The **HOLY SH!T** Moment

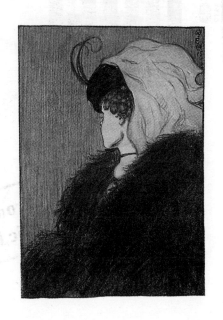

The HOLY SH!T Moment

How Lasting Change Can Happen in an Instant

JAMES FELL

Thorsons

Thorsons
An imprint of HarperCollins*Publishers*
1 London Bridge Street
London SE1 9GF

www.harpercollins.co.uk

First published in the US by St. Martin's Press 2019
This UK edition published by Thorsons 2019

1 3 5 7 9 10 8 6 4 2

© James Fell 2019

James Fell asserts the moral right to be
identified as the author of this work

A catalogue record of this book is
available from the British Library

ISBN 978-0-00-828868-6

Printed and bound in Great Britain by
CPI Group (UK) Ltd, Croydon

MIX
Paper from
responsible sources
FSC™ C007454

This book is produced from independently certified FSC™ paper
to ensure responsible forest management.

For more information visit: www.harpercollins.co.uk/green

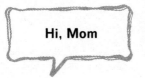

CONTENTS

Preface   ix

Introduction: The Librarian Who Put Down the Cigarettes
and Picked Up a Sword   1

PART ONE: EPIPHANY AND COGNITIVE BEHAVIOR CHANGE

1 The Antidote to Despair: The Euphoria of the
  Life-Changing Moment   25
2 Embracing Chaos: Quantum vs. Linear Behavior
  Change in the Role of Epiphany   53
3 You, Part 2: Finding Purpose via Epiphany   82

PART TWO: EPIPHANY AND THE EMOTIONAL SELF

4 What's Going On in There?: The Brain Science of the
  Holy Shit Moment   113
5 The Rock-Bottom Hypothesis: The Power of Epiphany
  to Battle Addiction   141
6 The Hand of God: Exploring Religious Epiphany   155
7 The Power of Love: How Passion for Life and Love
  Inspires Sudden Change   173

PART THREE: HACKING EPIPHANY

8 Dreamers Aren't Doers: Making Positive Fantasies
   Work for You Instead of Against You   193
9 Nudging Toward the Leap: Battling the Status Quo
   and Preparing Your Mind for Epiphany   212
10 Shamans, Drugs, and Rock and Roll: External Assistance
   in the Reevaluation of Reality   234

Conclusion: The Love We Found   246
Acknowledgments   249
Notes   251
Resources   269
Index   271

PREFACE

Psychology is not an exact science.

It is a field that Sheldon Cooper from *The Big Bang Theory* would deride for its lack of mathematical verifiability, and he'd be right. After all, when Sigmund Freud was pulling stuff out of a lower orifice to describe the "anal stage" of psychosexual development, Albert Einstein was creating theories of the universe that remain valid to this day.

Humanity's understanding of physics allows humans to build rockets that only sometimes explode. Our understanding of psychology allows us to . . . uh . . . wait.

It's not as bad as I allude to, but it is a discipline in flux. *Homo sapiens'* neurological processing unit is complex and beyond our current understanding of mathematical formulae to neatly explain.

When I first approached the life-changing epiphany as an idea for a book, I expected it would be a water-cooler "Hey, check out this interesting information" variety of tome. Like a Malcolm Gladwell book, but with swearing and the occasional mention of poop.

I never imagined it could be a "how-to."

But the more I researched, the more realistic the idea became. I gathered studies and spoke to smart people. I tried it on myself and my clients. I wrote articles and received enlightening responses.

There are no guarantees in life, but there is often good advice based on data and experience. We may not know all regarding the complexities of the mind, but human motivation has been studied for millennia. We do understand some interesting things, and through trial and error, people have transformed their lives for the better using myriad methods for change.

It turns out, the hare can kick the tortoise's ass when properly inspired.

Sometimes the slow-and-steady approach doesn't take you nowhere fast, it takes you nowhere at all. Conversely, the rascally rabbit has the finish line in its sights and is dashing toward it, invigorated, undeterred, unstoppable.

Finding true meaning, uncovering your real self, revealing your life's purpose—such things rarely happen via baby steps. These are transformations *unleashed,* suddenly, to great effect. Often, there is a "Holy shit!" thrown in to celebrate the momentous realization. The epiphany drives you forward, passionately pursuing the newfound aim. And great thinkers across the ages have interesting ideas about how to make such an experience happen.

Read on, and perhaps it will happen for you.

THE LIBRARIAN WHO PUT DOWN THE CIGARETTES
AND PICKED UP A SWORD

One cannot leap a chasm in two jumps.
—SIR WINSTON CHURCHILL

I saw *Jaws* when I was seven.

Children were free-range in the 1970s. Parents did their own weird thing that decade, so my sister and I got dumped at the local theater with regularity. It was a small town with one screen. In the summer of '75, it was a movie about a megatoothed murder fish or nothing.

I wish I'd sat outside and watched dandelions push through the pavement. To this day, I can't snorkel without hearing the music.

Despite living in the middle of a forest, after seeing the film I had nightmares that a great white was out to get me. A year later, the low-budget land-based knockoff, *Grizzly,* made my sleep even more of a horror show. My young brain could rationalize that hundreds of miles of spruce trees between me and the nearest ocean was even better than having "a bigger boat," but what about a bear?

He could be outside my window. He might be pissed about the bear my dad stalked, shot, and skinned, now a rug lying in the living room of our house. The grizzly might be seeking revenge on the only son of the sonofabitch who slaughtered his sibling!

"MOOOOMMMMM!!!"

I came within fifteen feet of a bear while out for a run a few years back and managed to not pee myself. Statistically speaking, I'm far more likely to die on the toilet, and I love my toilet.

I love bears too. I grew out of the fear and realized what amazing creatures they are, so long as you're not watching one rip Leonardo DiCaprio's Oscar-winning face off. You don't need to pack up your shit and head off to the great outdoors and have your own face-to-bear experience. I like imagining them because, as a metaphor, they represent that which is fierce and powerful. A grizzly is something with claws and teeth. When they are of a mind to do a thing, they are unstoppable. Also, like me after a long run, they don't smell too good.

When I imagine something kicking a lot of ass, I imagine a giant bear. And so when I have a lofty goal in need of chasing, I awaken my inner grizzly.

There is a grizzly bear hibernating within you, waiting for a key to unlock it from its cage. I want to help you find that key.

You have seen such an unleashed beast manifest in others; they become inspired about achieving their dreams and are relentless in the pursuit. My dad worked outside year-round and had the Grizzly Adams beard, but Mom was the one who let the huge furry quadruped loose. After the divorce, she moved us to the city and went all *Revenant* on glass ceilings.

Are there ceilings in your life you wish to burst through? Let's rattle that cage and see what we can stir from its slumber.

How you direct this powerful creature is up to you. As a health-and-fitness columnist whose work has been read by millions, and as a weight-loss coach, I first became aware of the phenomenon of sudden and dramatic life change regarding people's desire to change their bodies. But this is not a weight-loss book.

Okay, it's a little bit of a weight-loss book.

If you want it to be, it is. Because such accomplishments have cascade effects. Improving one's body is challenging, and those who attain the drive to do so rarely stop there. I've witnessed them go on to enhance their careers, improve relationships, conquer addiction, or undertake a complete life overhaul. Once the grizzly is free, there is no telling what adventures it will take you on.

That's enough about bears for now. Let's talk flying reindeer.

The Gift of Sudden Inspiration

"Growing old is mandatory. Growing up is optional."

My father says this often, as an explanation for his lovable goofiness. One day, I heard some motivational douche on the radio say those exact words, but as an imperative. His tone negative, the speaker proclaimed you must *work* to *grow up*, so you can be a *big success* or some shit. I don't know. He was trying to suck the fun out of life. Anyway, he totally came across like "I will death murder the shit out of your inner child!" and then I was like "Yeah, go screw yourself; my dad is cool and you're not," and I changed the station.

That inner child. Remember when you were a kid and believed stuff?

The Tooth Fairy and Easter Bunny are stupid, but Santa Claus? He kicks ass. There is a reason we let go of the Tooth Bunny earlier than the red-suited flying-reindeer wrangler: Santa is too cool to not exist.

I want to tap into your inner child, so you can believe some stuff. I want to tell you something so Christmas-Day awesome, you might have difficulty believing this present under the tree is real.

Except it's real as puppy breath. I'm going to science this baby up with a heap of evidence to show you. I'll share both far-out stories *and* studies about unlocking overarching awesomeness that takes life to a new, this-is-who-you-were-meant-to-be level.

You want big change? You want to be a badass at life? I'll tell you something about what it means to be Evil Gluteus Maximus. Or . . . no. I won't. Self-improvement is something that happens on *your* terms. *You* decide what is and is not the "Person You Were Meant to Be Registered Trademark."

Who is this person? Start imagining now. Take a moment and reflect on life experiences; couple them with your inner child. Dream big. Realistically big, because not everyone gets to be an astronaut. But imagine what you could do if you were suddenly inspired to *strive* for it. If you had the passion and drive to go on an ambitious quest, what would that new life look like? Not just the body, but the whole life: career, relationships, finances, happiness, self-worth, personal identity . . . Take a moment; take three moments. Invest some mental energy. *Think!*

You've heard it's about the journey and not the destination, right? Whatever. Despite what I just wrote, I'm not going to talk journeys too much in this book. Instead, *we are zeroing in on the moment your passion to take that journey is unleashed.*

Does this word "unleash" make you think of a process that happens slowly, step-by-step, through careful deliberation? Hell, no. It's a big-ass rottweiler straining to get off the chain and go fang-first into Nickelback.

It's when suddenly life—or the universe, or whatever—sends you a powerful message for which you cannot help but proclaim, "Holy shit!" at the revelation. (Profanity optional.)

I don't care if you believe in Santa or Satan, a golem or Gollum, an Indian elephant or Indiana Jones. Activate your imagination, and do some scientific discernment while you're at it, because we're about to take a voyage into explaining why you've been taking the approach to life change all wrong.

It may seem wishful thinking, what I'm about to tell you, but it's not.

We're about to unleash some shit.

Eye of the Tiger

I awoke at ass o'clock, guzzled some weapons-grade dark roast, and headed out for a six-mile run in temperatures hovering around hideous below zero.

As the sun rose, I did not lament the lack of sunglasses. They fog in under a minute at −20 degrees. Rather, my eyes were protected by a thick coating of frost collected on my lashes. Upon returning home, I snapped a selfie of my snowy visage and posted it to Facebook. The comments collectively proclaimed, "Dude, you are an entire cave full of batshit."

My pre-epiphany self would agree.

In a previous life, I abhorred physical activity, guzzled English brown ales, and stuffed McDonald's into my maw as though the apocalypse were imminent. Additionally, I was in debt, flunking out of college, and feeling like an unmotivated and out-of-shape bag of poo. But one day, the ground shifted beneath my feet. There was a transformative moment: a sudden strike of awakening in which my existence was split in twain; it became the instant that divided my life into "before" and "after."

Everything changed that day. Not that day—that *minute*. Those few seconds.

I have often said someone won't change their life in an instant unless they believe God threatened to shove a lightning bolt up their ass if they didn't alter their path. Divinely inspired or not, what I didn't realize at the time was how common the phenomenon of electricity in a posterior orifice can be for motivating rapid transformation. While coaching countless readers on the merits of the slow-and-steady path to change, I'd forgotten that wasn't how I'd done it. When I asked for similar stories of people who, in a single instant, found an overflowing fountain of desire to change their lives, I was amazed at the response. As I will show, research reveals that *sudden and overwhelming* motivation to change is more common than not in those most successful at it. This book contains many such stories.

Stories like that of Lesley Chapman, who picked up a sword, and her life changed.

Eleven years later, Lesley felt no pain. There was no dripping sweat, no aching muscles, no heart ready to burst out of her chest, and no lungs rasping like an asthmatic Darth Vader after a road trip with Cheech and Chong. No fear, either. There was only this moment: the fencing match of her life, fueled by adrenaline and a competitive spirit her old self wouldn't recognize.

The depressed, booze-chugging, overweight cigarette aficionado was no longer there; a lean and energized forty-four-year-old athlete questing for gold replaced the woman she had been. The new Lesley was a force to be reckoned with.

But her opponent was so fast; she struck like an arrow.

It was the last day of May 2015 in the city of Markham, Ontario, a multicultural community, part of the Greater Toronto area. The newly constructed Vango Toronto Fencing Center, located twelve miles north of the iconic CN Tower, was hosting the Canadian-American Veterans Cup, featuring the best fencers over the age of forty from across North America.

Lesley traveled from her home in the small town of Madison, New York, to take off to the Great White North for the first time, to prove her mettle after more than a decade of dedication to her bladework.

"I'd had a really good day," Lesley said. "I went to the tournament without a lot of expectations." As Lesley won match after match, her confidence in her sword-wielding abilities grew, and so did her enjoyment of competition. She beat someone she didn't expect she would to get to the gold-medal round and was elated at the opportunity for a championship bout.

The match took place on the raised platform at Vango, the fencing strip reserved for the final pairings. Long and narrow, the strip runs along a white wall that is painted with a large Canadian flag. Lesley and the woman she would challenge, Jennette Starks-Faulkner, were the highlight as they battled for overall gold in women's foil. Chapman took no notice of the crowd. All her attention focused on her opponent. She was in a state of *flow*.

Cue *Rocky III* music. It was "Eye of the Tiger" time.

"She is built like a teenager," she said of Starks-Faulkner, speaking respectfully of her opponent's physical build and skill; Lesley was honored to have this chance to compete against the world champion. But there was also a desire to prove herself. Six months previous, the two paired off in Reno, Nevada, and Starks-Faulkner throttled Chapman 5–0 in under a minute. Such a crushing defeat can be hard for a warrior such as Lesley to swallow.

Chapman explained she would be happy just to get a couple of points on her opponent. But because Starks-Faulkner was so small and fast, Lesley would have to outthink her to stand any chance of not repeating their match the previous December.

"When she attacks, she's like an arrow," Lesley said of Jennette. "I knew when she came at me I had no choice but to get out the way." Back and forth they danced across the raised strip, blades ablur in an ancient test of skill that used to be scored with blood rather than buzzer. Lesley's mind raced on how to outwit her opponent's superior speed. The tactics she devised used the advantage of her reach, following up a retreat from her opponent's lunge with a counterattack using her longer arm.

Lesley watched Starks-Faulkner carefully, fencing defensively, waiting for her opponent to lunge. When the strike came, she beat a hasty retreat, just out of range of her opponent's foil, then countered the smaller woman's lunging blade and scored her first-ever point against the champion.

"'Holy shit!' I remember saying," Lesley recalled. She knew she was still not at her opponent's level but she wanted to give her a good fight.

In such a match, it is often said you don't win silver but rather *lose* gold. After a long-fought battle, the final score was 10–6.

Lesley Chapman won silver.

Clicking into Place

The seed of Lesley's silver-medal win was sown in 2004 in a single, life-defining moment.

"I had been sedentary my entire life," Lesley said. "I was a good student and had it in my head that you were either a brain or a jock and ne'er the twain would meet." This attitude had a negative effect on Lesley as she reached her third decade of life.

Lesley explained that she smoked and drank and would often eat an entire pizza for lunch by herself. Significantly overweight, she believed this was what life had in store. She'd become fatalistic.

Life sucked. She wasn't happy but wasn't seeking change, either. Life was a slow, downward spiral she felt powerless to prevent.

"When you're drinking too much and smoking and eating crap all the time, it's going to chip away at your happiness," she said. She became depressed because she wasn't doing anything with her life. Her routine was work, drink, smoke, watch movies, repeat.

But fencing changed all that. Quickly.

Lesley's story is one of finding a passion for a specific sport that challenged not only her body but also her mind. She was living in Lexington, Kentucky, and an Olympic-fencing coach began offering classes at the local Y. Lesley heard an announcement about it at the university where she worked, and thought, *Why not?* Fencing was the one sport that held even a modicum of interest for the librarian, as it seemed sophisticated to her. "Grace Kelly fenced," she said.

She found the sport intellectually engaging. "You're concentrating so hard that you don't realize you're winded." In addition to the Olympic-level coach and the mental stimulation, there was another instance, a seemingly minor event, Lesley remembers with clarity, that defined the next stage of her life.

Many embark on a path of lifestyle change and suffer through for a while, only to quit, but not Lesley. What made her experience different? Why was her journey of personal transformation successful when so many others fail?

The answer can be found in a single moment, when a new sense of purpose clicks into place.

Lesley had been fencing just a couple of months. The fencing area at the Kentucky YMCA is an intimate space atop three flights of stairs; climbing them was a workout all by itself. She'd be gasping and sweating by the time she reached the top, wondering, *Why the hell am I here?*

Her commitment to continue was tenuous. Then a switch flipped.

On that day, early in her fencing career, Lesley noticed a group of child fencers had stopped their practice to watch the adults engaging in partner drills. Knowing she was being observed by these impressionable youths, she doubled her efforts at parries and lunges, trying her best to make a good show. "Suddenly, I felt like I belonged there," she said, "and that I wanted to get really good at this." There was a powerful awakening in both heart and mind that this is what she was meant to do. "In that emotional moment, I knew I would keep coming back to learn everything I could." It was an overwhelming sensation that made her feel as though she could weep with joy at what she had discovered: she would *not* quit. She would do whatever it took to become the best she could be. *She would not quit.*

Sacred excrement!

Suddenly and with surety of purpose, Lesley changed. It was not the step-by-step process like many behavior-change theories focus on. It was both instantaneous and total. A new part of her mind opened; a new Lesley was born, one that would never have to struggle to be motivated again.

She saw progress in her skill in increments, and it led to quitting cancer sticks so she didn't cough up alveoli during matches, giving up booze so the hangover didn't feel like she had a brain aneurysm during practice, and eating healthier to fuel performance and lose forty pounds so she could move faster and present a smaller target for her opponents.

"The changes are substantial," said William Miller, an emeritus professor of psychology and psychiatry at the University of New Mexico and co-creator of the popular behavior-change technique called motivational interviewing. Miller is also the coauthor of *Quantum Change: When Epiphanies and Sudden Insights Transform Ordinary Lives*. He is a leader among the handful of researchers examining the topic of sudden and massive psychological change.

For the book, Professor Miller and his coauthor interviewed fifty-five people who had experienced life-changing epiphanies to create a structure around the phenomenon. He explained there can be focal changes, such as ceasing an addictive behavior, adopting a physical activity, or even a massive shift in mood, such as dramatic alleviation from depression. But such sudden change can also be broad-sweeping—a total shift in identity with far-reaching impact through a person's life. What's more, his coauthor did a ten-year follow-up and found something incredible: "No one had gone back to their state before the event happened. To the contrary, everyone spoke of moving ahead."

Maintenance of the new behaviors, Miller explained, was high because it wasn't a struggle to do so. "People didn't talk about it using motivational language," he said. They changed at a fundamental level. They became a new person for whom the new behaviors were the norm. It's not a decision, it's a sudden transformation.

I remember my holy-shit moment, when everything became clear. It's when your inner grizzly is released from its cage as a roaring beast ready to achieve your utmost potential. It can manifest in various ways and for a multitude of reasons, but the reality is, *it happens!* It happens all the time—Professor Miller asserts as many as one-third of people experience such life-changing events—and yet we ignore the possibility of it happening for us. Accepting the verifiable reality of this phenomenon is the first step in making it happen for you.

It happened for Lesley that day, years ago. She was still overweight, still smoked and drank, and she was still a rookie fencer possessing negligible skill, but in that instant of self-reevaluation, her true personality awakened and ultimately led her to the silver-medal win. Along the way to a much healthier body, this new sense of purpose alleviated her despair.

"I decided in that moment that I was serious about becoming an athlete," she said.

The pounds fell off.

Escaping Quiet Desperation

Think of all the people throughout history who never had the chance to reveal their genius. Across the eons, most of humanity remained uneducated, toiling at physical labor to survive.

Henry David Thoreau wrote, "The mass of men lead lives of quiet desperation." Women too. Women *especially*.

But times are a-changin'. Bob Dylan doesn't want you to sink; he is telling you to start swimming. To quote from the Pixar film *Up*: "Adventure is out there!"

You have one shot at life, and it's not over yet. Many will continue to log the days, months, and years until they begin the long, slow slide into a dirt nap, heart songs remaining unsung.

For this to work, you must desire more. You must *thirst* for adventure. You must be ready to rattle the cage of the inner grizzly bear and yell, "Wake up! It's time to kick ass!"

Adventure can take myriad forms. Think of Lesley. Fat, drunk, inhaling cancer sticks, depressed, and going nowhere except continuing an unexceptional life, few if any marks made upon the world, no quests undertaken, no major life missions accomplished.

And picking up a sword changed all that.

As you read this book, I want you to continue to remind yourself that adventure *is* out there. Never in the history of bipeds walking the earth has there been greater opportunity to seize the day and kick its ass.

Start imagining now. The adventure begins in the synapses. Awaken the part of your brain telling you the path you're on isn't enough. Endeavor to find out who you truly are and the stuff you're made of. Embrace creativity in this mission. No one imagined the old Lesley as a champion fencer. Just because the astronaut spaceship has sailed doesn't mean there aren't out-of-this-world opportunities for you to chase.

Think of all the days since you came into the world as part 1 of your life. Your job is to imagine a lofty, exciting, purposeful path of You, Part 2. And just like *Star Trek II: The Wrath of Khan,* the sequel is going to blow away the original. As we move together through the chapters of this book, that's a big part of your job: creating a basic outline of this exciting sequel to the first part of your life.

My job is to awaken the power that inspires you to live it.

Daydream Believing

You may want to write this down.

Or . . . maybe . . . you don't.

I can't remember phone numbers worth shit anymore. That's because I don't have to. Used to be, I could glance at a number in the phone book, walk over to the phone, and *dial* it in. Not tap or punch. Dial. I'm that old.

Unless you're a troglodyte, you know that's not how we do it anymore. Now I can't remember seven digits without repeating them a few times; I'm out of practice.

A 2011 study published in *Science* reveals Google has a negative effect on memory, and as we'll learn, information gathering—cramming a bunch of stuff into memory—is an important part of inducing a life-changing moment. The study reports: "when people expect to have future access to information, they have lower rates of recall of the information itself." For these purposes, that's not good, because your brain needs to ponder things, twist them around a bit, and reorganize them in a way that makes sense. If your deep thoughts are consigned only to a notebook, your unconscious won't be examining them.

"Having a notebook is fine, as long as these ideas also stay in your head," said Mark Beeman, professor of psychology at Northwestern University and coauthor of *The Eureka Factor*. Beeman, who specializes in the neurology of creative thinking, explained that for generating a sudden insight, problems need to be turned over in your mind. And if a notebook takes these thoughts out of your brain and onto paper, it's counterproductive. Conversely, if the act of writing imprints them upon your synapses, or you are meticulous about revisiting your notes to examine such musings, then perhaps it's worthwhile. But a 2014 study published in *Memory & Cognition* says it might not help. Comparing two separate groups playing the card-matching game Concentration, the study found those who focused on memorizing did far better than those who made notes and then had the notes taken away.

For the course of the activities recommended in this book, I advise forgoing writing down every little thing in favor of pondering it, looking at new ideas from different angles using only your brain, and committing them to your gray matter for integration into solving of the problem *What do I do with the rest of my life?*

This isn't about achieving the answer via steady, linear analysis, but about having massive insight suddenly pop into existence.

I don't jot down such thoughts unless it's to log a specific idea I wish to write about. For examining your life and what the future must hold, however, specificity isn't usually the way. Beeman explained that for life-changing insight to strike, you need to have *all* the pieces of the puzzle floating in your brain at once.

It may take a while to gather enough information to achieve epiphany, and that's okay. There is time: time to daydream, time to imagine the new course. Whenever you're feeling pensive or have a few moments to envision the future stages of your life, engage in some free association and contemplate what possible paths you could take.

You don't have to go it alone.

Talk it over with friends. Surf the internet. Log on to social media and see what other people are doing. Wheels need not be reinvented. Seek inspiration from others who have been where you are.

Perhaps consider fencing. It's fun.

Take it all in, move it from the front of your brain to the back, then to the middle; put it on cerebral spin cycle for a bit, return it to the front, and see what gets spit out.

Sometimes a walk in the sunshine or an evening lying under the stars helps with the process.

Carved in Stone

You want to be like Lesley? Patience, grasshopper. Sudden change in one's motivational level may happen in a moment, but the stage must first be set. Evidence reveals that you can stack the deck in your favor and *make* epiphany happen.

As a test, I made a significant one happen for myself while researching this book. There is an important aspect of my life I have tried to change many times, over years and years, always to no avail. But then I used some of the methods outlined in this book, and that was it. The desired change happened. I *made* the ground shift, and a major life change took place just like that. *And it was easy!*

That story is in chapter 10. This was not a small thing like making my bed every day or flossing my teeth. It was much bigger, and I have reaped tremendous benefits from the experience.

I want to help you get there, to reach the point where a new sense of purpose awakens and your unstoppable will is unleashed. To do that, you need to understand the phenomenon of sudden transformation, so you can open yourself to possibility.

For Lesley, in that single moment of fencing practice, when she felt her sense of belonging and purpose awaken, her life altered course and gave her the power to keep altering it. This is the secret so many who change their bodies, break addiction, and achieve success and happiness often miss: To change their lives, they first must change their sense of who they are. The concept of shifting one's identity is a recurring theme in *The Holy Sh!t Moment,* because that's what epiphany does: it doesn't change behaviors, it changes you.

The traditional methods of behavior change preach the tortoise approach over that of the hare, but there is a problem with that story: The hare in

Aesop's fable was an idiot. If he'd been smart, he would have kicked that reptile's ass.

When it comes to changing who you are, sometimes it's better to be a hare. It is an amazing thing to experience a potent, emotional event that shocks you into clarity of purpose. Besides, baby steps are lame. Why slowly build a bridge across that chasm when you have the power to leap to the other side?

This instant transformation of will seems magical. But sometimes you must meet the magic moment partway.

I had a life-changing epiphany that arrived out of nowhere, and it spurred me to action, to go from flunking my courses to acing them, as well as to getting out of debt. That accomplished, I tackled my physique next, and that part was, shall we say, less inspired for a time.

I had to do the traditional baby steps. I had to be the tortoise. I had to slog.

But not for long. My mind had learned to recognize epiphany. Over the course of two months, my attitude shifted from "This sucks" to "This isn't completely horrible." And realizing that regular exercise no longer felt like a soul-destroying endeavor initiated a massive and rapid transformation of mind-set. I put in some hours and met the magic moment along the way.

As did Lesley. Remember, her life-changing epiphany didn't happen the first time she held a blade. It took a couple of months of parries and ripostes to awaken a sudden and total transformation into who she was meant to be.

You will read of others in this book who did *not* have to meet epiphany partway. Lightning struck out of nowhere, and they were inspired from day one. That totally happens, and I hope it happens for you. But if it doesn't, you're going to have to be ready to do some uninspired work while keeping your brain attuned to receiving inspiration. In coming chapters, I'll offer advice on using traditional methods of step-by-step behavior change to help generate a sudden leap forward.

There are myriad methods of rapid and significant life change, but all such roads share one undeniable characteristic: a deep emotional sensation that carves a new sense of purpose into a person's being, like a chisel working on stone. Conversely, the traditional (read: boring) models of gradual, step-by-step cognitive behavior change seem to be lacking in their ability to create passionate adherence. Resultantly, such laborious methods of struggling to develop new habits may not be the most effective way of achieving change.

Sometimes *dramatic* lifestyle change "just happens" because of reaching enlightenment that arrives *beyond cognition.* Again, this is not a decision; it is an *awakening.* Such an awakening inspires one's determination and dedication to succeed.

Sometimes Santa Claus does exist, and he brings you a gift of overwhelming passion to kick ass at life.

And such sudden change is a scientifically explainable phenomenon one can pursue with purpose, leaving less to random chance, to create a better life. This book is about providing you with actionable tasks that help set the stage for a specific moment: that space in time when something so vital and important takes place inside the mind that your life is divided into "old you" and "new, righteous, unstoppable you."

It's the moment the grizzly is released from its cage. Suddenly free, the massive beast looks you in the eye, tilts its head back toward its massively muscled back, and says, "Hop aboard, kid. You and I are going places."

What Is an Epiphany?

I have a couple of master's degrees and am a stickler for the science. This book includes references to reams of peer-reviewed journals alongside exclusive interviews with some of the most renowned experts in behavior change on the planet.

That's why it pains me to use Wikipedia as a reference.

From the ancient Greek *epiphaneia,* meaning "manifestation, striking appearance," an epiphany is often described as a scientific breakthrough, or religious or philosophical enlightenment. However, it can represent myriad situations in which deeper understanding is suddenly attained.

The apocryphal story of an alleged apple falling and allegedly hitting Sir Isaac Newton on the head describes when he allegedly had an epiphany about the nature of gravity. Alas, this is not how innovation and techno-logical advancement work.

In his book *The Myths of Innovation,* author Scott Berkun's first chapter is titled "The Myth of Epiphany." In it, he describes the story of Newton and the apple to debunk the popular understanding of epiphany. The author then quotes the primary inventor of the laser, Gordon Gould, to provide an example of how scientific advancement *usually* works.

> *In the middle of one Saturday night . . . the whole thing . . . suddenly popped into my head and I saw how to build the laser . . . but that flash of insight required the 20 years of work I had done in physics and optics to put all the bricks of that invention in there.*

A pot-smoking teenager watching *SpongeBob SquarePants* in his parent's basement isn't likely to have a stroke of brilliance regarding the nature of light amplification. Gould, a renowned physicist who had worked on the development of the first atomic bomb, spent twenty years of toil working to resolve an enigma, and when enlightenment was finally achieved, some would refer to that as an epiphany. But it is no such thing. It is simply that last piece of the puzzle—a puzzle he'd been working on for decades—being put into place.

Human behavior can work in similar ways. One may have been debating, mulling over, and gathering information about a new path for years, and a life-changing event—that triggering moment—is the final illumination before they are ready to make that sudden switch from unconsciously "thinking about it," to an instant and wholehearted *This is happening!*

Conversely, it truly can strike out of nowhere, because decisive behavioral change is not often the same as building a laser or theorizing gravity. It can be as simple as hearing an old song on the radio. You may be driving along, listening to the classic rock station, and Van Halen's 1992 hit "Right Now" comes on and you *feel* it; you realize it is indeed your tomorrow, and you decide to catch the magic moment. Such a phenomenon can reshape your sense of being and purpose in life in a near instantaneous wave of emotion that provides you with new insight and motivation regarding the way forward.

Lesley Chapman didn't dwell on what was wrong with her life or how to change it until that singular moment when she discovered what it was like to feel something *right*.

For some, they need to hit rock bottom before they're ready to leap toward the light. You don't need to be that desperate, but you're reading this because you know that change—be it moderate or massive—is something you desire. If you feel dramatic change is something you *must* achieve, then you also need to seek out a transformative moment to initiate such change.

Much of the pre-work involves information gathering and embracing new ways of thinking, but it also requires not letting sudden insight pass you by.

It involves opening your mind, asking the question *Is this it?*

It's about looking at the world with an investigative mind-set, in which what you seek is opportunity to change. Inspiration can arrive from *anywhere* and at *any time*. Be prepared.

Is. This. It?

Ask yourself that question when you experience something that *might* be a catalyst for change. Most of the time, the answer to the question is going to be "No, it really isn't." But it's all practice.

It can be because of this practice, the opening of yourself, the attunement, that allows epiphany to strike. Speaking of practice, getting stuck is good.

"When you tackle a problem, and fail to solve it, it sticks in your craw—and your brain." This is from Professor Beeman's book *The Eureka Factor*, coauthored with John Kounios, a professor of psychology in cognitive and brain sciences at Drexel University. The authors explain that ideas can require an "incubation period." The work you do thinking now doesn't mean you have your epiphany right now too. You work until you "get stuck." Then the unconscious takes over while you're busy doing other things.

In most stories of major life transformation, an epiphany is almost a constant. Many who have experienced massive change can identify a specific instance when their outlook got on track in a much more positive way. Changing one's body is a powerful manifestation of the moment of change, because a healthy body often equates to a healthy mind, and overcoming the challenges associated with physical improvement also imparts valuable life skills. I mean, unless it's weight loss resulting from unhealthy methods such as popping unregulated diet pills like they're Skittles or going on some batshit crazy fad diet some celebrity is flogging. The latest dietary dumbassery I heard about was an Oscar winner proudly proclaiming the completion of her eight-day-long, goat-milk-only cleanse. I'm happy I don't have the job of cleaning her bathroom.

The Snowball Effect

There is a switch inside many people set at "I can't."

When it flips over to "I can" for one thing, it doesn't stop there. Research shows life-changing epiphanies are rarely "one and done." Often the catalyst for initial change is a massive mental shift, but smaller epiphanies can arise at random during people's life journeys, to bump them further along their quests to be the best humans they can. Professor Miller explained that people who have such experiences often have further, clarifying epiphanies later in life. "There appears to be an opening to having that experience," he said.

Take a moment and think back: *Has this happened before?*

Have you experienced a life-changing moment in the past? What was it like? How did it manifest? Can you relive it? Can you imagine something like that happening again? Did you learn something important from the experience you can bring toward future life change?

If the answer is yes, it's called a "past performance accomplishment." It's a parameter of self-efficacy theory, created by Stanford University psychology professor Albert Bandura in 1977. It's about how you form perceptions regarding your ability to perform specific behaviors. Past success = confidence, which makes people more determined to persevere, even in the face of adversity.

If you've had an important insight in the past, it makes it more likely you can have one again in the future. Cue Jimi Hendrix: *Are you experienced?*

Positive life change can assume myriad forms; don't fret if you're not interested in pushing your body. But I do encourage contemplating some form of activity as part of the new you. I say this because you were not meant to sit idly and watch Earth spin on her axis. You were meant to rise and join the fray that is the human condition. Movement empowers from top to toenails; it can even come to define you, should you find the right exercise.

Whichever activity a person chooses, if they enjoy it, is the right one. The path ahead has more choices than there are beers in a Munich autumn. Finding which flavor suits best requires taking a few taste tests.

The Holy Sh!t Moment is about achieving the clarity of purpose to carve your own path to success.

Switching Tracks

Consider this word carefully: "momentous."

The topic of this book is not about merely *deciding* the future path your life will take. It is about a *momentous event* in which you suddenly become aware of *the answer* and change at a fundamental level from the experience. It's not only a spark of insight, it's an awakening of passion.

Such an "answer" is rarely well-defined or black-and-white, and effort is required to find your way along the appropriate path.

Do you remember *The Karate Kid*? Not the worst film ever, but the message is dogshit.

Perhaps you're too young, or maybe you were there, in that theater, and you disagree. That's because it was the eighties, the decade of bad decisions, even though we didn't realize it at the time. So many pastels . . .

Go ahead and watch it again—the original with Ralph Macchio—and see if you realize why the message it relays is canine feces.

My wife is a second-degree black belt in karate. Both our children are black belts, and my daughter competes at the international level. I can attest that you don't get good at karate by spending a few weeks waxing cars and painting fences. You get good at it because it's your lifelong passion.

And because it is your passion, *you are motivated to do the damn work, hours of work, day after day and year after year!*

The Karate Kid disrespects the work by advocating an extreme shortcut to success. It disrespects the fact that my daughter has been in karate since she was five years old, and trained her ass off, sometimes twenty or more hours a week, to win that gold medal at the USA Open ten years later.

Work is glorious, and inspired work transforms. It transforms your body, your mind, your spirit. Someone who kicks ass at life is not a sofa-sitter. Such people can be efficient, but they're not the type always questing for a quick fix. They don't believe—using weight loss as an example—that some miracle macronutrient ratio is going to open a rift in the space-time-insulin continuum and magically transport their belly fat to a parallel universe. They *know* effort is required, but they don't mind, because they've become inspired.

Work equals accomplishment, the forms of which can be innumerable, and such accomplishments are habit-forming. Again, this is far from being just about diet and exercise. For someone who feels their life lacks purpose, it can be an amazing thing to suddenly find more drive than you know what to do with.

Here is a quick task. It should only take a few seconds, but that doesn't mean it will be easy. You ready?

Make a promise to yourself that you're done with believing in bullshit quick fixes and unrealistic shortcuts to major accomplishment, be they accomplishments with your body, your brain, your career, your finances, or your relationships. Accept reality: it is *work* creating your desired outcome. Do it now. Integrate this fundamental truth. Then move forward.

The overarching goal is to change the way you *feel* about the work so it doesn't seem like work. *That* is an attitude adjustment that can happen in just a few seconds. There *can* be a rapid change in mind-set. You can't become a karate master quickly, but you can become *inspired* to do it in an instant. It's this accelerated mental shift that has the power to change your life.

As British historian and philosopher Arnold Toynbee said, "The supreme accomplishment is to blur the line between work and play." Your passion to achieve can be triggered in that single defining moment when you realize, *Enough of this bullshit.* Motivation is no longer a scarce resource after such a momentous event. It comes built in.

Being active is hard. Eating healthy is hard. Conquering addiction is hard. Relationships are hard. Making money and advancing your career is hard. *Life* is hard, whether you choose to work at improving it or not. A life-changing moment can make everything much less of a challenge. Sometimes, if the epiphany is powerful enough, it makes the changes not just easier but mandatory, because every new step feels as though it was meant to be. The recipient of the epiphany is *compelled* to walk this new path, perhaps even race down it.

Speaking of racing and things that are hard, recall the words of President John F. Kennedy regarding the space race and putting a man on the moon. He said we choose to do these things "not because they are easy, but because they are hard."

You should aspire to do more with your life.

Because it is hard.

Act Now!

- Dream (realistically) big and imagine the new person you want to be.
- Think of an ambitious quest you could undertake.
- Develop a thirst for adventure. Remember the librarian who traded cigarettes for swords.
- Consider not using a notebook, but instead committing ideas to memory for regular rumination to achieve later enlightenment.
- Ponder until you "get stuck." Then engage in a diversion to let your unconscious continue working at it.
- Endeavor to meet the magic moment partway. Realize you may have to engage in some uninspired work prior to the lightning strike.
- Become attuned for lightning to strike. Ask yourself, "Is this it?"

- Ask if a life-changing moment has happened to you before. Examine if this is something you have experience with— determine if you have a past performance accomplishment— so you can use that knowledge to make it happen again.
- Accept that work is not only necessary but glorious in its ability to inspire passion and transform you. Try to find work that will feel like play.
- Remember the words of JFK and embrace change: because it is hard.

PART ONE

Epiphany and Cognitive
Behavior Change

THE ANTIDOTE TO DESPAIR:
THE EUPHORIA OF THE LIFE-CHANGING MOMENT

There are opportunities even in the most difficult moments.
—WANGARI MAATHAI

On the schoolyard field of battle known as gym class, I made the geeks look good. I was such a klutz, I was always picked last when teams were selected. I often came out of dodgeball with head trauma.

In college, I got the "freshman fifteen"—those pounds one tends to put on during their first year—factored by three. I was twenty-two and felt my life was circling the drain. As mentioned before, my health, finances, and scholastic situations were a mess. There was no fall from grace; my life had always been blah, and it was my fault.

I wasn't just a bad athlete growing up, but a bad student. I was smart but lazy. I squeaked my way into an easy postsecondary program with half a percentage point to spare, then promptly began failing. I went to the campus pub instead of class. The credit-card companies were calling. Things were bad and looking worse; I was about to be kicked out of school because of my poor grades.

I was in a hole of my own digging; Joan Baez pulled me out.

The folk singer's words appeared in the school newspaper, and my life changed in a moment.

"Action is the antidote to despair," the quote read.

I sat in the food court at my alma mater, reading the comedic highlights of the paper's section referred to as "Three Lines Free." It's a place for students to publish quotes and witticisms and proclamations of undying love or temporary lust. Partway through reading, Joan smacked me in the face. It was so simple to realize that, as bad as things seemed, they could be fixed via concerted effort.

In that instant, my life switched tracks.

Because, you see, there was a woman.

Her name was Heidi. I loved her like no other. You know stories of finding "The One"? This is such a story.

She was a straight-A student destined for medical school; I knew flunking out spelled the beginning of the end. I say this not to ever speak ill of her. But you must know that she, an amazing woman, deserved a good man; a man I had yet to become.

I was in a state of despair, and taking action—working hard for something for the first time in my life—was the antidote.

And suddenly I felt so much better. Even though no effort had yet been expended, the *anticipation* of having these problems and this beer belly no longer weighing on me was euphoric. It's like when you hear your parole has been approved and you're getting out of prison but you're still in prison. I've never been to prison. I got some speeding tickets when I was younger, but I paid them. Anyway, euphoria and stuff . . .

Instead of hitting the pub as I'd planned for a few barley-based beverages to wash down a plate overflowing with fries and gravy, I got up and booked an appointment with the appeals committee to beg my way out of my failing report card, allowing me to continue as a student. It was the first step of many, and it felt right.

When it comes to experiencing a life-changing epiphany, the way things feel is critical. It involves, as mentioned earlier, unleashing one's inner quadruped.

The concept began with the classical Greek philosopher Plato. In the fourth century BC, Plato wrote a "dialogue" titled *Phaedrus,* which contains an allegory about the charioteer. In it, the driver of the chariot represents a person's more rational self, the guiding force based on intellect and reason. (Because those guys doing the death race in *Ben-Hur* were totally reasonable.) Conversely, the horses pulling the chariot represent a person's emotions; they are what provide the power to move forward. And if they want to run wild, the driver of the chariot can do little to control them.

Let's ignore the part about Plato's horses having wings, so as not to confuse the issue.

It is important to note that the horses are not like-minded. According to Plato's tale, one is more virtuous in its passion; the other has a dark side driven by baser appetites. One wants to train for a marathon; the other wants to down tequila shots then go in search of a chili cheese dog to later throw up.

The goal of the charioteer is to obtain the help of the noble horse to overcome the desires of the troublesome one. Otherwise, you're blowing your groceries in the gutter. I've done that. It's not fun.

The allegory was adapted some millennia later, in 2006, with the publication of *The Happiness Hypothesis* by New York University social psychologist Jonathan Haidt, who referred to the rational, conscious mind as the "rider" and increased the size of the emotion-driven, unconscious-mind quadrupeds to a solitary elephant. Part of the upgrade involved increasing the intelligence of the beast, asserting elephants are smarter than horses. As we'll see when we examine the neuroscience of attaining sudden insight, Haidt is right. In most cases, the unconscious driver is the correct one; the conscious needs to learn to listen.

A short time later, the rider-vs.-elephant analogy became a core component of the 2010 book *Switch: How to Change Things When Change Is Hard*, by brothers Chip and Dan Heath. Chip is a professor of business at Stanford, and Dan is a senior fellow in entrepreneurship at Duke.

A determined elephant will go where it pleases, regardless of the urgings of a more rational rider. To achieve a desired destination, one must appeal to both rider and elephant.

The elephant is the passion and the drive. Whereas the rider may prevaricate and overanalyze, the elephant is the part of the human spirit that can change directions in a flash, and with powerful determination, because it is driven to get shit done. Rather than needing to ponder, it is *compelled to act.*

Let's try an experiment in which you talk to your four-legged friend.

How do you *feel* about changing?

In the introduction, I asked you to awaken your thirst for adventure. I expect you generated some ideas of songs unsung, mountains unclimbed, finish lines uncrossed. And now you're faced with the opportunity to sing your way across that finish mountain, or something. Have you got it? It doesn't have to be concrete. Big picture is fine for now. Is it in your brain? Are you thinking about it?

Good. Now stop.

Stop thinking.

Instead, start feeling.

Don't *rationalize* this change. Don't try to think about all the reasons why you should stop doing a thing (like sitting all day, drinking too much, smoking, being angry, overeating treat foods, doing drugs, staying in a dead-end job or relationship, wasting money on stupid crap) or start doing a thing (going back to school, exercising, eating healthier, being kinder, working at your career, spending more quality time with loved ones).

I want you to stop thinking, because of paralysis via analysis. If these goals you imagine—things to stop and things to start—have been around in your brain for a while, you've already thought them to death. And yet here you are. Still struggling. You rationalized your way out of change. Well, crud.

Time for a dramatic change of tack.

Ask yourself: *How do I feel about this change?* You don't completely cut thinking, but alter the focus. Instead of thinking about this new path, you're examining your emotions. It's not about making a list of reasons why and why not. It's opening your mind to what your heart is saying, metaphorically. I know the heart doesn't literally control this. It's still in the brain, just a different part. Enough semantic blather. Let the feelings flow and listen to what they tell you.

Why are you reading this sentence?

You're supposed to be examining your feelings. Examine your change! You go feel it now. I'll wait. I'll even put an extra space between paragraphs to make it easier to pick up again.

Welcome back. How did it go?

Was there a twinge? Did you have a moment? Was there a positive rush of emotion? Did you gain some special insight or wave of motivation to change because you quested to understand your *emotional* drivers rather than rational ones?

Was the grizzly released from its cage?

Don't fret if it didn't happen. We just began and will work through exercises like this at appropriate times throughout the book. And hopefully lightning will strike.

Hopefully.

There are no guarantees. But the harder you work at these exercises, the more you strive and the more you *believe* epiphany can happen, the greater the likelihood it will.

It's like that song by Journey, the one about the mythical place called South Detroit we've all heard way too many times: "Don't stop believin'."

It's in your head now, isn't it? My bad. But take something good from it.

Believe. Believe it's possible to unleash your beast. In *The Eureka Factor,* Kounios and Beeman write, "Insights are like cats. They can be coaxed but don't usually come when called." You must learn to coax your elephant. Or grizzly. Or a really determined kangaroo, if that's your thing.

Conscious thought rarely incites life-changing epiphanies. Instead, the snap revelations to change in a moment are based on what is often an over-whelming *feeling* that it is right, arriving from the unconscious. As Plato and subsequent authors revealed, it is such an emotion that gives epiphany its power. I was in fear of losing a beautiful and brilliant woman who let me see her naked, and I felt quite emotional over the impending loss of love. She was not threatening me in any way, but I knew deep down that such a driven woman (she had a perfect GPA and completed medical school at the top of her class) wouldn't stay for long with a drunken dropout who was letting his health go to hell.

I got my shit together, and we made babies. Told you she was The One.

Beyond ancient philosophy and its modern interpretations, we have the scientific insights of Nobel Prize winner Daniel Kahneman. Known as the Father of Behavioral Economics (which we learn more about in coming chapters), Kahneman, an emeritus professor of psychology at Princeton University, is the author of *Thinking, Fast and Slow.* The "fast" way of thinking is the elephant. It happens when an unconscious idea pops into consciousness. It can also be that emotional driver one needs to effortlessly change. Kahneman refers to this as "System 1," writing that it "operates automatically and quickly, with little or no effort and no sense of voluntary control." Conversely, "System 2" is the rider. It "allocates attention to the effortful mental activities that demand it, including complex computations."

Kahneman explains that System 2 is where we make our rational choices, our conscious decisions. His description is telling: "Although System 2 believes itself to be where the action is, the automatic System 1 is the hero of the book."

You're damn right it is. System 2 is the supporting character, and an inherently lazy one at that. Kahneman writes that System 2 engages in the "law of least effort." But that doesn't mean it's useless in this regard. Far from it. As the Heath brothers explain in *Switch,* you have to appeal to both elephant *and* rider. Kahneman says System 1 constructs the story, and System 2 *believes it.* System 1 "is the source of your rapid and often precise intuitive judgments." It is a "mental shotgun" allowing us to answer, in an instant, those tough questions about our lives.

Time for a wee task.

I thought about calling these tasks "Action Items," but I didn't want you to have a full MBA Bingo card by the end of the book (being that I have an MBA, the risk is real). *Implement these Action Items to proactively synergize an optimized epiphanic paradigm!* Just, no.

Give us a kiss. Except all caps: KISS. I've interviewed both Paul Stanley and Gene Simmons. Paul is nice. . . .

Man, my System 2 is all over the place right now. KISS = Keep It Simple, Stupid. A 2011 study published in *Personality and Social Psychology Review* looked at "feelings as information." The study asserts feelings are a "sensible judgment strategy," but don't overthink it, especially in terms of the advantages of change. That's because when you create a comprehensive list of all the benefits of something, the study showed, it becomes less appealing. This is System 2 overanalyzing what System 1 came up with. Your task is to not let that happen.

When System 1, the fast-acting hero of your life, says, "This is it!" the supporting character of System 2 will come up with a couple of confirming rationalizations as to why, yes, we can agree that this is likely the thing. Then *STOP!* Once you have that confirmation, just go with it. You don't need to keep drilling down into the benefits, or it actually becomes less compelling. This doesn't apply to using System 2 for *enacting* the vision. Being detail oriented in that regard is important.

The Gap between Thinking and Doing

"All the world's a stage, and all the men and women merely players."

William Shakespeare wrote of the stage and players and how life is one big performance in a monologue from *As You Like It*. But the speech also refers to seven stages of a person's life.

I only know of this play because it was quoted in the 1981 hit song "Limelight" by my favorite band. Beyond that, I possess mere high school knowledge of Montagues, Capulets, Macbeths, and whatever the last name of that Danish lad was, the one who pondered if he should be or not.

Speaking of Hamlet's act 3, scene 1, soliloquy, crossing the gap between thinking and doing *is* making the decision to "take arms against a sea of troubles, And by opposing end them."

You may be facing a sea of troubles, but what could your life look like if you took up arms and charged fearlessly ahead, fierce and furious in your determination to take not a single prisoner but emerge victorious?

Hamlet's oft-quoted scene begins with, "To be, or not to be?" At the darkest period of his life—dad dead due to the dastardly deeds of his dick uncle—the young Danish prince ponders his future actions, struggling with the decision that lay before him. Should he accept his outrageous fortune, or get in its face?

Oh, wait. It's Shakespeare. Everyone dies. Bad example. Let us move back a space to the moment *before* the decision to take arms was made. Some centuries after Shakespeare laid down his mighty pen, James Prochaska, a psychology professor and director of the Cancer Prevention Research Center at the University of Rhode Island, developed a different model for the stages a person goes through when experiencing life change.

Along with his colleagues, Professor Prochaska developed the trans-theoretical model (TTM) of behavior change, which is one of the most studied lifestyle transformation models ever created. Since its initial development in the 1970s, more than $80 million and 150,000 study participants have contributed to its peer review. It's no longer used much for designing psychological interventions, but it's still useful as an examination tool.

There are five stages to TTM:

1. **Precontemplation**—People in this stage are not even thinking about altering their behaviors, as they do not see their current lifestyles as problematic. *This couch is ever so comfy. Never shall I remove my bottom from its padded glory and proximity to the rectangle of glowing time waste.*

2. **Contemplation**—This is when a person is thinking about changing their behavior, but not quite ready to act. *Hmmm. Is there such a thing as a "couch sore"? Perhaps if I repositioned a little. Dammit, I emptied the DVR of all the good stuff. Is there anything new on Netflix? I suppose I could go outside. . . .*

3. **Preparation**—In which the person is focused around planning for acting toward behavior change, which is intended to be imminent. *Outside it is! I just need to wiggle myself out of this massive ass groove I've created in the couch first. . . .*

4. **Action**—When a person is engaged in behavior change. It is a challenging time, when fragile habits are formed. *Later, couch! Fresh air, bitches!*

5. **Maintenance**—In which habits from undergoing the action stage are more ingrained and the new behavior becomes sticky as the person gains self-confidence in their abilities. *What's a couch?*

Under the TTM model, where is the lightning strike? Where does the critical moment that divides a person's life into before and after take place? We can see it in the gap between thinking and doing, between stage 2 and stage 3. It happens after contemplation and before preparation. Although the stage that follows is called "Action," preparation is still a form of doing, a form of action. It is a giant leap forward toward a new life, which happens in an instant. It requires bravery and force to leap this chasm; hence the need to ensure that the emotional grizzly-elephant-horses are shocked into wakefulness and pointed in the right direction. They have taken up arms, roared defiantly, and the sea of troubles trembled at the might of such a battle cry.

Sometimes the movement from contemplation is a mere step, but that's not what you're after. What you seek is a giant leap. Because if this moment that prompts the advancement to stage 3 is a powerful one, if it is a true epiphany that enlightens and inspires, you'll have little fear of relapse.

The new behaviors stick.

The Decisional Balance Sheet

"Reaching a tipping point to move toward action involves a change of focus," James Prochaska told me. "One goes from the balance favoring the 'cons' of adopting a new behavior to giving more weight to the 'pros.'"

Unfortunately, people tend to slide back into old habits, which is why it is important to ensure the decisional balance sheet is well stacked in favor of acting.

"A person is going to be a lot better prepared to stick with the new behavior if the pros *significantly* outweigh the cons," Prochaska said. If the pros only slightly tip the balance when you start down the path to changing your life, you will still be experiencing those cons. If you *just barely* decide to change—if, exasperated, you throw your hands in the air and say, "Fine! I *guess* I'll do it"—you're going to *feel the suck* of that change; it can overpower any benefits. The balance teeters around ambivalence; you are more inclined to give up and slide back into old behavior.

In 2010, Jennifer Di Noia, a professor of sociology at William Patterson University in New Jersey, worked with Prochaska on a meta-analysis of twenty-seven different studies of how TTM was used to evaluate decisional balance; they were specifically looking at dietary changes to affect weight loss. Published in the *American Journal of Health Behavior,* they came to some fascinating conclusions.

During the precontemplation stage, cons rule the synapses, but something interesting happens during contemplation: The balance begins to shift. And it shifts in a way that explains why so many fail in their efforts to change their lives.

In the contemplation stage, the reduction in thinking about cons is small; the balance shifts because the value of the pros increases by a significant margin. The cons are still there, still powerful. The fear of pain or boredom from exercise, the financial worries over pursuing a different career, or "You can peel my wine glass from my cold, dead hand!" remain palpable. And to overshadow such fear, the pros need to "Hulk Smash!" them into insignificance. The ratio revealed in Di Noia and Prochaska's research of pros to cons is enlightening. They discovered the pros must *outweigh* the cons by almost a *2 to 1 ratio to be truly effective!*

It stresses the importance of the great leap forward achieved via some form of epiphany; it's not a simple tipping of the balance sheet to 51–49 in favor of the pros. Again, it's not a small step forward toward successful and sustainable change; it works better if you take a giant leap.

"Pros and cons of decision making is not a conscious, rational, empirical process," Professor Prochaska said. "It is very emotionally based."

What can make someone passionate about a new direction? What gives them the drive to charge ahead with an unstoppable "no-prisoners" attitude? Prochaska explained that a dramatic event could cause someone to reevaluate pros and cons.

Such a dramatic event found its initial spark for Chuck Gross in January 2008. He sat in an Irish pub in New Orleans, called Boondock Saint, having a quiet beer or five. The bar was named to pay homage to a cult-action film of a similar name.

"My brothers-in-law are twins. My wife and I took them barhopping on Bourbon Street for their twenty-first birthdays," Chuck, a computer programmer in Pittsburgh, told me. The Irish-style pub was dark and somewhat gloomy. A mirror advertising Guinness hung on an aging brick wall. Being it was a twenty-first birthday event in the French Quarter of New Orleans, Chuck was in no shape to walk a straight line.

That night, Chuck had a chance meeting that would be the first step on a journey that would change his life.

"Back then I was not a social person, being as fat as I was," Chuck said. He described two seats at the far end of the bar, and how he ended up sitting next to an average-looking man who practically forced Chuck to speak with him.

The man was in his fifties, clean-shaven, plain-faced, and wearing glasses, Chuck recalled. His hair was gray-white, he had an outgoing personality, and it seemed like he couldn't help but engage in conversation. Because Chuck had consumed a few drinks, he began to loosen up.

The two men talked for a time of things inconsequential, and then the man informed Chuck of his profession as a photographer, which he proclaimed gave him the ability to read people. "I see the fear in your eyes," the man told him.

Chuck admits that his memory was hazy due to alcohol consumption, but insists the stranger never brought up Chuck's weight. Rather, the man told him he could see there was something Chuck wanted to do, and that the fear he felt soon wouldn't be a problem in this quest.

Chuck Gross was taken aback that a random stranger would speak to him in such a way. I advocate against poking one's nose into the body weight of others; people should mind their own business. Even though Chuck's obesity was not mentioned, it was obvious what the man was talking about. The conversation ended abruptly but still had a profound effect.

Two months later, Chuck Gross was dead.

Lightning Strikes

The life-changing epiphany seems rare because people aren't forthcoming about it.

William Miller and his coauthor write in *Quantum Change*: "people who experience such events are often reluctant to discuss them openly." In their research, they uncovered that many had told only one or two people, and some never told anyone. I'm kind of a big deal on Facebook, so when I asked, people came forward.

Bragging over one's social-media following is the epitome of pathetic, but if you want to "Like" my page, it's facebook.com/bodyforwife.

During the interviews, Miller and C'de Baca write, "the words came tumbling out like a great unburdening." Yep. That's what happened with my interviews, too. It's because such an event changes how people feel, what they think, how they experience the world. It is a Big Deal. Life will never be the same.

Freaked out a little right now? I mean, Chuck Gross died, right?

It's a good kind of lightning strike, however, like when Luke learned he was to become a Jedi, except without having your aunt and uncle burned to a crisp by Imperial Stormtroopers.

Of the fifty-five people interviewed for *Quantum Change*, the authors explained that for 80 percent of them, it "took them completely by surprise." And for half, nothing special was happening leading up to it. This reinforces Beeman and Kounios, who say lightning strikes during diversion after getting stuck.

To repeat: keep working at it, follow the steps in this book, then take a break and let the unconscious do its thing.

Let's get back to Chuck.

As forward as the stranger's words were, it nudged him from the pre-contemplation stage to the edges of contemplation. Cons of change became slightly minimized, and pros garnered more investigation and emphasis.

"During those two months, the conversation was eating away at me both subconsciously and consciously," Chuck said, explaining that many of the things one experiences when they are that heavy are buried because they're constant: back pain, aching feet, always being out of breath. Before, they were facts of life, but after the meeting, he became more aware of them. Chuck's brain was becoming primed for lightning to strike.

It was March 11, and the Pittsburgh winter edged toward spring, a time of rebirth. Rather than forget his chance meeting at Boondock Saint the previous January, Chuck dwelled on it.

Then it happened.

"My wife Denise came out of the bathroom with a positive pregnancy test," Chuck said. He explained this was not something planned for. They'd talked about having children, but it was always for the future, when he was healthier and had lost weight.

"The lightning bolt was instantaneous," he said. It first hit him with overwhelming joy that he was going to be a father, but he also knew with absolute clarity he had to do something about his condition. He described it as though someone hit him in the back of the head with a baseball bat, full swing.

The bat to Chuck's skull was what ended his life, metaphorically speaking. "I tell people I died that day. The old Chuck is dead. I killed him."

Chuck's realization that he had to change happened in an instant, when he knew he had to become not just the father his child needed, but the husband his wife deserved. Yet Chuck didn't stop thinking there. The powerful "Aha!" moment brought additional clarity to who he was and how he needed to change.

"I realized that a big part of my identity was wrapped up in me being fat," he said. The emotion of the moment was clear; years later he struggled to tell the tale. Voice thick, Chuck explained he was always the fat kid growing up; people made fun of him for it. His identity was as the funny fat guy; the guy girls wanted as a friend, but never to date. People knew him for being able to eat and drink a lot, and that was all. With the pregnancy announcement, Chuck had a new identity thrust upon him, that of a father, making his values pivot hard in a new direction.

In 2016, researchers from the University of Oregon published a study in *Psychological Inquiry* about the "identity-value model" of self-regulation. The authors theorize that "behaviors that are connected to identity are more likely to be enacted because they hold greater subjective value." They examined the dieter's dilemma, investigating how people struggle with eating healthfully, and how self-control is about two opposing processes: impulsively eat the doughnut, for example, because it's yummy, or strive to regulate that behavior and resist the treat in favor of vegetables?

When someone's identity is one that places high value on healthy eating, there isn't much struggle. It's not a matter of exerting willpower; it's acting in a way that is in direct relevance to *who they are.* At the beginning of this book, I mentioned awakening the grizzly, but it's more about *becoming* the grizzly.

The final part of Chuck's process to destroy that old identity and create a new one involved stepping on the scale. Technology lent him a hand.

"The scale was only rated up to 400 pounds and always gave me an error message, but this time it worked and read 410." That's what made it real; it reinforced for Chuck what he had to do. He needed to embrace the identity shift.

Chuck described hating exercise; he hated watching what he ate, hated trying to lose weight only to fail again and again. "Before, I never felt like I'd be able to change." But this time was different. This time, it was not the rational thought prompting him forward, but a new sense of being filling him with emotion. That lightning strike / baseball bat to the head doesn't come from a considered weighing of the pros and cons; it's an overwhelming sensation in which an internal spirit awakens and proclaims: *This will happen!*

Chuck's transformation was so total that I had no idea of his amazing story when I first met him in 2015. It was at a fitness conference in Kansas City, in a hotel room after-party. I assumed he was another fitness aficionado and was surprised when he replied to my call for stories. We met again in 2017 and 2018 and shared a big hug each time.

I told Chuck's story to Michael Inzlicht, a professor of psychology at the University of Toronto and a longtime critic of the idea that willpower is some depleting resource we need to ration in order to change behavior.

"Chuck sounds like he had this experience that didn't change his self-control," Inzlicht said. "He changed his identity." Being a good dad was something Chuck would hold in high value, and this was the identity push he needed because of his concerns about his ability to be active with his children and even live long enough to see them grow. As a result, "The value of losing weight dramatically increased."

Chuck described his old identity as an anchor that needed to die for him to move forward. This was the defining moment that divided his life into before and after. "The person I am now was born that day," he said.

From ashes gray, a phoenix arose.

But what does this all mean? How did this one moment help Chuck lose over two hundred pounds and keep them off? The first part to understand is that insight, driven by emotion, unlike rational analysis, is something possessing the power to crush doubt.

"There was an overwhelming sense of joy and relief," he said. "I didn't need to struggle with my motivation; it came built in." Chuck described a sense of inner peace; there was no question he would do it. There were still struggles to overcome, but he had momentum that began that day; it pushed him forward.

I want to repeat something Chuck said, because it's damn important. Let's bold, italicize, and center it to draw attention:

"I didn't need to struggle with my motivation; it came built in."

This is what we're going for, dear reader. *Right there* is the reason I'm writing this book. Dropping over two hundred pounds and keeping them off takes tremendous effort, but having it feel like *destiny,* that you have an endless fountain of desire to achieve, after years of trying and failing, can only be attained by a sudden, transformative experience. I'm not saying amazing accomplishment can't be attained by way of baby steps, but that way sucks, and the failure rate is high.

Rapid transformation of desire to succeed is *so much cooler!* Wouldn't you rather do it that way?

Maybe not. Maybe that identity-shift stuff freaked you out.

But I want to alleviate that fear, because you're going to change anyway. We are, all of us, changing all the time. I'm quite a bit different from the man I was ten years ago, and *way* different than the one from twenty-five years ago. While a life-changing epiphany is something that feels like it is something that happens *to* you, the preparatory work, along with your life experiences and deepest desires and understanding of your true self, help ensure it was something coming *from* you. This isn't an outside agency acting upon your brain; *this is your brain.*

Yes, if this happens, you're going to change. A lot. Quickly. Sounds scary, but it comes with an overwhelming feeling of *rightness*. And that's why it drives you. We'll examine the neuroscience behind this shift in coming chapters, but for now I ask you to trust in the power of your unconscious and conscious processing systems to find the correct path.

Time for another mental activity.

Think of what happened to Chuck, and *why* it happened. The overwhelming epiphany seemingly came out of the blue—but did it? The seed was sown back in that New Orleans bar. He became more aware of the negative consequences of his current path. He also talked with his wife about how children were for "later," when he got healthy.

And then it all came crashing down in an instant with a pregnancy announcement. Chuck received an overwhelming vision of the man he *must* become, for his wife, and for his unborn child.

Chuck was suddenly "pro" focused.

The cons of changing didn't matter; all that mattered was *becoming.*

Your next task is to maximize the pros. Imagine one or three of the things you'd like to do. Create a basic vision of the You, Part 2, that I spoke of earlier.

Now imagine what it's like to be that person.

Focus on just a few of the major benefits you will receive from this change. As I showed earlier, don't overanalyze, but ponder some of what will be awesome about that new career, new body, new location, or new life. What are the big things that make it so desirable?

Are these good things not just good, but amazing? Are they *inspiring*? Do they make you desire this change so much that you *must* achieve them? If not, perhaps the problem is you're not being ambitious enough in your vision. But don't be so ambitious that you choose an objective which is unachievable.

This is called the "expectancy-value approach," a behavior-change theory dating back to 1967. It dictates that we engage in those behaviors we both *expect* to be successful at *and* have high value to us.

Think on this: What kind of benefits would it take to inspire you to action? Merge this with consideration of the feasibility of the goal. You can still dream big, because implausible does not mean impossible.

Create another vision. Think of a new you so incredible it becomes irresistible. Push the boundaries of realism. No one gets to be Batman except Batman, but you can still achieve awesome. There's only one Wonder Woman, yet you can become a wondrous woman.

What does the limit of your potential look like? More important, how does it feel to imagine the benefits of standing in those shoes?

Don't expect this will cause lightning to strike now. It's information for percolation. But it might happen soon, so be ready, just in case. A transformative moment *might* happen in chapter 1, or it might happen in chapter 9. It might happen three months after you finish this book. Work the problem until you're stuck, engage in diversion, and you could have a transformation like Chuck did.

Chuck went from despair to joyous determination in an instant. *Joyous* determination. This sense of elation Chuck described is a parameter of the transtheoretical model called "dramatic relief." It can take place when one moves from the contemplation stage and into the preparation stage, from thinking to doing. It is because the *anticipation* of resolving one's weighty problems generates a sense of euphoria. You're like, *Hell, yes! I see light at the end of the tunnel now, and I will run toward it. Nothing will stop me.*

How does the feeling last? What keeps you on the new course, besides the shift in values and identity? The secret is in the synapses.

James Prochaska explained that such dramatic relief could involve either negative or positive arousal. Positive arousal involves being inspired to chase something good. But negative arousal, unlike the name might imply, is not a bad thing: it's about removing a negative feeling, such as conquering an addiction.

I was in a state of despair, and taking real action, working hard for something for the first time in my life, was the antidote. In that moment, I understood that solid effort could change everything. The *enlightenment,* the realization that I was *about to take action,* cured my despair that day, and step-by-step, progress was made toward a new and better life.

The emotional arousal from a momentous epiphany is like a hit of a powerful drug, and it is because pleasurable neuromodulators are activated. A new path is created in the mind, and each step forward in that better direction provides a little rush of positive reinforcement that whispers, *This is right*.

At a simple level, how these neuromodulators work for ongoing motivation can be described via operant conditioning, as outlined by psychologist B. F. Skinner early in the twentieth century. It's stimulus-response; the epiphany is such a positive experience that every additional step taken (the stimulus) that stays true to the vision allows the recipient of the vision to continue to feel that sense of rightness from its pursuit (the response). More details are in chapter 4, but it's this neurochemical boost that makes you take the next step, and the next one.

The quest comes to rule the synapses.

Self-Compassion vs. Self-Loathing

If you hate your body, you'll be less inspired to change it. Because passion for health rarely comes from a place of self-loathing. Same goes for hating your life.

There are those who lose weight because they were filled with disgust over their bodies. It can work for some, but research indicates shaming and self-loathing over obesity leads to comfort eating and immobility far more often than generating action.

In a 2013 study, researchers at Florida State University assert that not only does stigmatizing obesity lead to poorer mental-health outcomes, but the authors state, "Rather than motivating individuals to lose weight, weight discrimination increases risk for obesity."

And a 2003 study by University of Texas at Austin psychology professor Kristin Neff revealed the importance of self-compassion in boosting one's psychological function. It "involves being touched by and open to one's own suffering, not avoiding or disconnecting from it, generating the desire to alleviate one's suffering and to heal oneself with kindness."

It contrasts with efforts to boost self-esteem, which have come under criticism. Self-esteem often means judgments and comparisons, evaluating personal performances in comparison to a set of standards, as well as examining how others view you. And while low self-esteem can have negative psychological outcomes, boosting it is not a panacea for the psyche. The first issue is that it's hard to raise, and the second is that targeting self-esteem can lead to self-absorption and even narcissism.

Part of the benefit of focusing on self-compassion is that it's not just about you. It "represents a balanced integration between concern with oneself and concern with others, a state that researchers are increasingly recognizing as essential to optimal psychological functioning," Professor Neff wrote. Winning at life need not involve competition. You may have a sudden insight that the best thing for your future is to dedicate yourself to helping others. Look at Chuck. He wasn't thinking about looking in a mirror or strutting on a beach. He wanted to be a good dad.

We will examine self-compassion meditation techniques in chapter 9.

The body is often a source of one's self-loathing, so I'll share the words of Taryn Brumfitt, a body-acceptance advocate and director of the documentary film *Embrace*. She told me of the need to not descend into negativity: "I have never met a single human being that has made lifelong, meaningful change that came from shame or guilt." Conversely, she has seen much positive change resulting from self-care, self-love, and self-respect. "I'm asking people to embrace their positive qualities."

I gained a lot of weight in my early 20s and I hated myself, but the harder I tried, the less possible it seemed to lose weight. Finally gave up in my 40s. But then something clicked. I decided I needed to be kinder to myself, love the body I had, and love what it could do. Before I knew it, I had the confidence to get a trainer. . . . I feel the best I've felt and looked in years!
—*Victoria*

I bring this up because all this talk of unstoppable desire to succeed and motivation and willpower can send the wrong message.

Sticking to weight loss as the example, we live in an environment that manufactures body fat. With over two-thirds of Americans being classified as having excess weight or obesity, and the fact it happened in a few decades, it's clear there has been a major societal shift contributing to it.

Obesity is not a personal failing. It's not a choice people make. It's not something to be ashamed of. Just because this book is about exploring the mystery of generating a massive leap in motivation does not mean those who don't experience it are somehow lesser.

Losing weight or changing your life in other ways is complex. That's because human motivation is equally complicated. A big problem with the weight-loss industry is a lot of the strategies are built on suffering, which are not effective for the long term. People feel the failure is their own rather than due to a corrupt industry that failed them.

I spent years unhappy with my weight. . . . I would hide food and opt out of gym whenever possible because I had been told so many times at that point that my body was flawed, I didn't believe it was capable of anything. . . . In my late 20s, joining the body-positivity movement helped me see value and worth in my body and what it's capable of . . . and I will be completing my 4th half marathon next month. —Amanda

You may have an epiphany that you're done with worrying about your weight and decide to focus your energies on things more important to you, and I am 100 percent cool with that. It's your life; you have the power to choose your own road.

If you're guilty of beating yourself up, it's time to ditch the self-loathing and accept yourself for your faults and your capabilities. Use your newfound self-respect as part of the process to energize your desire to find the best way forward for you.

Accept your humanity and that all humans are flawed. Being a perfectionist gets in the way of self-compassion. There will be detailed steps later, but for now, endeavor to ditch shame and guilt, and, in so doing, try to better understand yourself. Take some time to analyze what makes you unique. What are your strengths? Where do your capabilities lie? What could you accomplish if you were truly determined? Why would you be able to accomplish these goals? What is it that *you* bring to the equation that makes these goals attainable? Focusing on your qualities and your potential, imagine what your post-epiphany journey might look like.

You need to know yourself better, because there is no cookie-cutter approach to creating an optimal life outcome. It is unique to you.

I like cookies.

Exceeding Expectations

There are people for whom life has been criminally unfair. The cards they've been dealt are a puddle of cat puke.

It is possible, dear reader, you are one such unlucky feline-vomit recipient.

When it comes to body weight, myriad factors can add fat to your frame: genetics, environment, finances, abuse, mental illness, medical conditions, medication. . . . Regardless of a dream of getting in shape and/or bettering one's life, there can be preexisting problems that will hamstring efforts.

People who proclaim anyone can achieve anything if they just work hard enough need to shut up and go far away, then shut up some more.

Life isn't fair, and because it isn't fair you must not feel shame or a need for comparison. Some have immense privilege. Others, their lives suck, and it is not of their own making.

And yet they are told to "Just do it." They are shamed for their weight and shown photoshopped models on magazine covers as the "ideal" they should aspire to. Beyond that, there are the societal expectations to have fancier cars, nicer houses, bigger paychecks, better-looking spouses, and smarter children.

I'm calling bullshit on all that.

This is about you and bettering *your* life by playing the hand you've been dealt to the best of your ability. Yes, you *can* achieve a great deal by being passionate and inspired to succeed; you can exceed all expectations not just with your body, but with your career, happiness, relationships, and more. But it is still worth comprehending the reality of your situation.

There is merit in aiming high, because if you only make it three-quarters of the way to your goal, you're still overjoyed at how much you've accomplished. But do not aim so high—do not quest for the unattainable—if failure to become Batwoman or Wonder Man would crush your will to continue.

Seek greatness on your own terms.

Fulfilling Life's Purpose

Lee Holland had a "sit-down job," something her family envied.

Living in Chattanooga, Tennessee, she came from poverty and was one of the few to finish high school and the first to go to college. She worked in a small cubicle as a customer-service representative for a major health-insurance company, which was seen as a big step up from working in fast food or doing manual labor. But her life felt unfulfilled, like she was going through the motions. Lee felt destined for more. All that was missing was the drive to figure out her purpose in life and then to chase it.

The drive arrived in fall 2007.

She took a call from a man who worked at a carpet mill in rural southeastern United States. He was calling because his young son had been diagnosed with a rare form of bone cancer. The man was so relieved because he had just been recalled to work after a layoff and had medical insurance again.

Unfortunately, Lee had to tell the man his policy had a "preexisting-condition clause," and any new diagnosis in the first year was not covered. This was prior to the Affordable Care Act, when the law changed, requiring policies to not have such restrictions for children.

Lee wanted to help. She had previous experience working for a state Medicaid contractor and saw a chance to get the boy coverage. She called the Medicaid office and was told they *would* cover the child, but only after they received a denial explanation from the insurance company Lee worked for. Prior to her company being able to issue such a denial they needed to send the boy to a pediatric oncologist. The problem was, the only such specialist within one hundred miles of the client refused to see the boy unless they knew they'd receive payment. Her company wouldn't cover them. Medicaid wouldn't guarantee payment until they received a denial explanation from her company. It was a catch-22: her company couldn't provide denial until the boy saw a pediatric oncologist, but the oncologist wouldn't see the boy unless payment was guaranteed.

But she'd done her job. In fact, she'd already gone above and beyond. Company policy was to end the call and move on to the next customer.

"At that moment, something in me broke," Lee Holland told me.

Not caring that it was against the rules, she blocked calls on her phone and walked into her manager's office. "I told him he could fire me at the end of the day, but I was going to get that child on Medicaid and in to see a pediatric oncologist." Her manager replied with, "Do what you have to do."

It required several phone calls, a discussion with her company's legal department, and signing of privacy release forms, but she got the boy approved for Medicaid and scheduled to see an oncologist by the end of the day.

It was all buildup. After her shift, Lee's life-changing moment came in the parking lot as she walked to her car.

It was a gray November day; a light drizzle fell. Then a question popped into her head: *What are you doing working in customer service when you can help people like this?* There was a sudden snap decision to change careers. It came so fast, she didn't even break stride as she closed the final steps to her car. "I didn't know what it was yet. It was just between me and the universe that I was going to do *something*. I felt I had potential to help people through the chaotic mass of the American health-care system." The realization, Lee said, was like a dislocated bone suddenly popping back into its joint.

"I had instant drive to do it," she told me.

The moment she got home she logged on to her computer to look at what education programs she would need. Thirty-six years old and possessing a degree in cultural anthropology, she began by upgrading her science and math courses at a community college. There were many challenges over the next decade, but for Holland, there was never any doubt she was going to make a difference in the world. She recently graduated with a doctorate in pharmacology and a master's degree in public health, and has accepted a research fellowship in D.C. that ensures pharmaceutical quality for Medicare and Medicaid recipients. She has won prestigious grants, awards, and scholarships, conducted important research, delivered numerous presentations, and mentored other students.

At first, Lee was leery of pursuing a doctorate as part of this new path in life, because it was a four-year commitment and she was already in her forties at that point. But a friend explained the time would pass anyway, and in four years she'd be four years older either with or without the degree, and her mind was made up. "There were a lot of challenges in between," Lee said. If one path didn't work out, she had to find another. "Even though I had suddenly become singular in my determination, I had to be flexible about the way I did it."

And it all changed in that parking lot in 2007. "Since then I've met so many amazing people. My social life exploded. I got to travel the world." She also met her husband and has been married for eight years.

"Now I feel like I'm really fulfilling my life's purpose."

Tuning In to Being Turned On

In the introduction, I discussed the "magic moment" and how you might need to meet it partway by engaging in traditional methods of behavior change for a while and hoping epiphany strikes somewhere along the way. It's also important to not let the magic moment pass you by. This is your final task for chapter 1: I want you to envision what it's like to *seek* the magic moment.

Lee Holland might have missed hers. It wasn't anything jarring like a sudden pregnancy announcement. She had done her job and could have ended the call, but in her mind, there was an opportunity to really help, to make a difference on that one day. She was somehow *attuned* to that opportunity, and it primed her brain for that epiphany in the parking lot.

Imagine what it's like to be attuned.

Now that you know a life-changing epiphany can come from anywhere, it's important to be able to recognize it. Yes, it is powerful; usually so much so that there is no denying the experience. But perhaps it needs a nudge. Perhaps it doesn't take place in a microsecond, but over several seconds. So instead of squashing down the beginnings of overwhelming emotion because you're too cool for that, imagine what it's like to embrace the feeling, explore it, and let it flow.

Because in the first second or two you could lose it by ignoring the sensation or even crushing it. Society conditions us to not show too much emotion, but screw that. You must feel this experience and feel it deeply. This book is about learning how to experience something so powerful it changes you down to the bone marrow. I want you to experiment with breaking with your conditioning and *seek*.

Seek meaning from your sudden insight.

Too often we tune out, seeking constant entertainment to distract from what our unconscious is trying to tell us. Break from that and examine these moments when the brain goes off on a tangent and, rather than try to snap out of it, explore it. Feed that sensation some fuel.

What kind of fuel? The kind that understands that, as humans, we seek experiences that allow us to be comfortable, and by attuning yourself to a life-changing insight, you must be willing to get uncomfortable. Lee had that comfortable sit-down job her family envied, and she knew that rejecting it to chase opportunity would involve struggle.

"One does not become fully human painlessly."

These are the words of twentieth-century psychologist Rollo May. In his 1950 book *The Meaning of Anxiety*, he wrote of how such negative emotions can be a good teacher, because while we can avoid the reality of certain problems, the feeling of disturbance is something we carry with us: it gnaws. Suffering, said May, is an integral part of growth. Take that pain, pull it like a sword from its scabbard, and *wield it!*

That being written, please don't go off your prescribed anxiety medication. This is just about using your negative emotions to spark personal evolution. Mark Beeman explained that anxiety triggers analysis, and analysis is the opposite of insight. But it's still part of the process. Remember: Work until you get stuck. Analyze, then engage in diversion. As we will learn later, it is during a positive mood when epiphany is most likely to strike.

This book is not all "Think positive and you can live your dreams!" ad nauseam.

There is an adage in motivational speaking and internet memes: "Dream it. Wish it. Do it." And it is bullshit, because this is not an easy road of endless happy thoughts in which if you keep your eye on the prize and always think positive, you'll miraculously attract what you desire.

You must rethink positive thinking.

Gabriele Oettingen is a professor of social and developmental psychology at New York University and the author of *Rethinking Positive Thinking*. She explained to me it's beneficial to have these lofty goals you wish to pursue, but not to daydream about your achievement, because it creates complacency. If you fantasize about how wonderful life will be after you've attained your goal, it fakes a sensation of already achieving it, so you no longer strive. Instead, focus on overcoming obstacles to achieving the goal. (Details on how are in chapter 8.)

Changing who you are can be frightening. As a concept, it may fill you with dread. But it's not some scary Jekyll and Hyde personality shift. You're still *you*, just an improved version. It's about change for the better, not worse.

When you learn to control fear of change, you open yourself to becoming more.

Priming Directives and Quantum Leaps

"Mount St. Helens blew up in a single moment."

Sherry Pagoto told me this as an analogy of a life-changing epiphany. She's a full professor at the University of Connecticut and a clinical psychologist specializing in behavioral counseling for obesity. "But the explosion was years in the making."

We may not even see the pressure building, but it doesn't mean it isn't there, simmering away, ready to explode like a Diet Coke with a dozen Mentos dropped in.

Thinking about the future is but one action helping prime a brain for change, Pagoto explained. Often, for people to be able to make a massive leap of behavior change, they must have been pondering it in some way. It can involve a feeling of malaise, depression, or dissatisfaction. Conversely, such thinking can revolve around a desire to improve, to transform from good to great. Such thoughts may reside in the back of our minds for years before we're ready to act upon them.

Contemplation can be subtle. It can build and build, but still, there is resistance to change because it is both fearful and challenging. And yet one day a time may come to pass when one cannot hold it in any longer and the emotional volcano erupts. A specific life event can bring it about. But what control do we have over these dramatic, triggering events?

That is not an easy question to answer, because life, and our approach to it, is often chaotic in nature.

Chaos theory can help us understand the dilemma better. A branch of mathematics examining complex systems sensitive to small changes in initial conditions, chaos theory has been referred to as the "butterfly effect," a metaphor that lets us imagine the minor air disruption of a butterfly's wings culminating in tornado formation weeks later. Slight alterations at an earlier juncture can end up yielding widely different results farther down the line in a person's life.

I first learned of chaos theory from actor Jeff Goldblum in the 1993 film *Jurassic Park*. While seductively placing droplets of water on costar Laura Dern's hand to show how minor alterations in initial conditions would affect which way the drop would roll, Goldblum explained that the theory "deals with unpredictability in complex systems."

The human brain is a complex system. *Life* is a complex system.

About those "minor alterations" in initial conditions: Subtle changes in where the droplet was placed or how Laura held her hand or even the way the breeze was blowing could cause the droplet to go in a different direction. Such is the case with life as well. What if Lesley never picked up a sword? What if Chuck and his family had chosen a different bar? What if Lee hadn't gotten that call? What if the person who decided to quote Joan Baez in the school paper picked Judas Priest lyrics instead? How would all our lives have turned out?

Such questions are difficult to answer because behavior change is not always a rational, linear process.

Sometimes it's a quantum leap.

Act Now!

- Take a break from *rationalizing* change and instead examine your feelings. Get emotional and listen to what it tells you.
- Remember that song by Journey and "don't stop believin'."
- Let the fast, intuitive System 1 be the hero, and make the slower, rational System 2 the supporting character. Don't let System 2 overanalyze the benefits of the story System 1 constructs. Get the confirmation, then stop.
- Forget worrying about the "cons" of change and instead imagine how powerful the "pros" will be. Endeavor to become pro focused.
- Again: Work till you get stuck, then divert and let the unconscious do its thing.
- Accept that this is about change both in identity and values, rather than a change in behavior. The altered identity-value construct makes new behavior adoption automatic. Lose the fear of becoming a new person, because this is a critical component.
- Aim high, but realistically so. Choose goals that have a high value to you but are deemed achievable via concerted effort.
- Embrace self-compassion. Don't hate yourself or what you see in the mirror. Realize positivity is the path.
- Don't daydream overmuch. Keep your fantasizing of achievement to a minimum so as not to sap energy. Rather, consider the primary obstacle to success and how to overcome it.

2

EMBRACING CHAOS:
QUANTUM VS. LINEAR BEHAVIOR CHANGE
IN THE ROLE OF EPIPHANY

A moment's insight is sometimes worth a life's experience.
—OLIVER WENDELL HOLMES, SR.

My grandmother was an evil and bugshit bonkers hell-beast of a woman who hated everyone and everything. A while back, we were having a family get-together, and my sister asked which kid had possession of grandma's engagement ring.

"Isn't that one of her Horcruxes?" my son said.

The joke slayed; 10 points to Gryffindor.

Speaking of crazy grandmothers and things that slay, there was blood everywhere, and I was screaming. The blood was pouring out of my left knee. Childhood trauma provides vivid recollection despite more than four decades having past.

We were visiting my grandmother in Victoria. A friend named Brent was chasing me through the house in a game of tag, and the sliding glass door that led to the back deck was sparkling clean.

In other words, I thought it was open. I *was* only five.

Fortunately, I did not go *through* the glass. I hit it with my knee and it shattered, then I fell backward, away from the shards. Blood poured forth from my knee as screams ripped from my throat in equal measure. This, followed by Uncle Jim driving me to the hospital through the rolling coastal hills at a speed that punished the suspension of the pre-1970s-model four-door car while my mother had a minor meltdown in the back seat as she attempted to hold my knee together with six squares of toilet paper.

I still hadn't stopped screaming. I remember the screaming, not the pain.

Thirty stitches plus an annoyed doctor and nurse later, we went back to Grandma's house, and she proceeded to chew me out about her shattered door.

That was my first inkling she wasn't such a nice person.

I achieved a fuller realization she was "cuckoo for Cocoa Puffs" a few years after destroying her window. My parents had split, and we had no choice but to live with her for six painful months. I was getting an apple and she told me to give her half. I got a knife and cut, and being a young lad, it was a haphazard job. I was left with one piece substantially larger than the other.

It seemed wise to give my grandmother the larger half, so I did. Then she proceeded to berate me for being a "greedy little bugger." She told me I should have given her the bigger half. I was looking at my half, which was about one-third of an apple, then looked at her two-thirds of an apple and said to myself *You really are a nutbag.*

I won't repeat any of the racist slurs she often spewed.

For three decades, I watched my grandmother torment my mother. My mother told me horror stories about her childhood, and I believe them. Mom had one of the shittiest, most abusive childhoods you can imagine. So, yes, she's a little neurotic as an adult.

But she is not at all abusive, quite the opposite.

I have never wanted for love. Mom showered my sister and me with love to the point it was almost annoying. "Yeah, I get it, Mom. You love me, but now you're embarrassing me." I always knew from my earliest days that, no matter what, Mom had my back.

And yet, when she became pregnant for the first time with my older sister, there was panic. My mom dreaded she would be like her own mother and perpetuate a cycle of abuse. She spoke of this to her doctor, who gave her some simple yet poignant advice: "The suffering you've endured can be undone by loving your children with all your heart. Think of what your own mother would have done, and do the opposite."

The advice sounded good but did not resonate. The fear remained.

Later, at home, she felt my sister kick. My mother told me of feeling the growing child inside her. She believed the kick was a message saying, *I am here, and I need you.* Even though my sister was not yet born, my mother realized in that instant she loved her in a way she had never loved another person before.

Her heart soared.

In a moment, she *knew* she would never be like her own mother. Down to her core, she was certain she would be the most loving and caring mom she could be. And she has been.

I'm not crying. You're crying. Shut up.

Such a sensation, in which you achieve total clarity of purpose in an instant, qualifies for the word "epiphany."

No matter which way epiphany manifests, you must listen. It's the path to a better life.

Speaking of a better life, my mom didn't let her upbringing hold her back. She earned her corner office in a male-dominated industry, becoming a business juggernaut celebrated in the community. What's more, she took a near-impossible high road with her own mother, continuing to look after her rather than write her off. She even forked out for a nice nursing home when the old bat lost the last of her marbles.

The lesson is this: The circumstances of the first part of your life don't have to define the second part. No matter what transpired yesterday or the days preceding it, this does not determine what happens on neither this day nor the days yet to come.

No one makes it through life without scars. Some are visible, like the one on my knee; others reside below the surface. Sometimes change happens fast via epiphany. Sometimes it takes years and baby steps. Change is inevitable, but you're the one who influences the direction such change will take.

If you're tired of the path you're on, you can switch to a new one. They're your feet, and you have the freedom to place them where you choose. A quantum leap of inspiration to change your path does not mean you lack liberty. Just because your new way forward has become irresistible does not mean you have sacrificed self-determination. Rather, your heart and mind being united in what feels *right* is what gives epiphany its power to push you.

When you feel such power, it means you are about to fulfill your destiny.

Off the Quantum Deep End

The word "quantum" is being increasingly used in health circles to the point that it is almost considered to be pseudoscience.

What I am about to write is not pseudoscience. It's Einsteinian science. And other kinds of real science. Quantum has been a real science thing for a long time and it's still a real science thing.

Ironically, I chose a science-fiction author to explain it to me.

Digital Decision-Making

The first time I met Rob Sawyer, I was worried he was about to die. Being we were not yet friends and that I am sometimes selfish, my initial concern was how this affected me.

Rob is a Hugo Award–winning science-fiction author. Early in 2005, I registered for a weeklong science-fiction writer's workshop at the Banff Center in the Rocky Mountains, to be led by Rob and taking place in September of that year. I'd read Rob's work and seen his photo on book jackets, and when I met him at a book signing four months prior to the workshop, he looked nothing like I expected.

He'd lost a *lot* of weight. So much so I was concerned he had a terminal disease. My baser self worried that if he died, there would be no workshop.

But Rob was happy and energized, and the workshop was a great experience that led to us becoming friends. The first book of his I read was titled *Factoring Humanity*. I recall the main character created a "quantum computer" that could process infinite calculations per second because it operated in multiple dimensions, or parallel universes, or something.

Now you know why I wasn't cut out to be a science-fiction author.

In addition to being a best-selling author (one of his novels, *Flash-Forward*, became a TV series on ABC), Rob is a sought-after speaker and futurist because of his ability to communicate complex scientific phenomena in lay terms. At the time of our conversation on the nature of quantum leaps, Rob was putting the finishing touches on his twenty-third novel, serendipitously titled *Quantum Night*. The fact that Rob had his own epiphany, which led to dropping a third of his body weight, a loss he has sustained for over a decade, makes his insight even more relevant. But before discussing his personal story, we spoke of the true, scientific meaning of the word "quantum."

"Most things in life go along in an analog wave; they go up and they go down and they change gradually and continuously," Sawyer said. He explained, when it comes to losing weight, the motivation for most is like that analog wave: sometimes it peaks, such as when the high school reunion is coming up, and other times it bottoms out, and the only desire is to braid one's ass into the couch and shove Doritos down one's neck.

With quantum cognition, however, there is no wave. "Quantum is not analog," Sawyer said. "It's not wavelike. It's digital. It's either on or off. It's either this or that."

This or that . . . these are the same words I heard from Def Leppard guitarist Phil Collen, who we'll hear more from later, when he spoke to me of battling his addiction. After a struggle with alcohol, Collen suddenly quit drinking at the age of twenty-nine. "It was very black or white," Phil said of quitting. "I knew I had to go this way or that way." (Note: It can be dangerous and even deadly to suddenly quit substances such as alcohol as well as benzodiazepines, more commonly known under names such as Valium, Xanax, and Ativan. Consult a physician.)

To reveal the science of the quantum leap, Sawyer went down to the atomic level. "We talk about the quantum leap of an electron, going from a lower energy state to a higher state." Sawyer explained that this doesn't mean an electron travels to that higher state the way a mountaineer ascends Everest. It's not step-by-step. It means the electron has gone instantaneously from the base of the mountain to the peak, bypassing all the intermediate steps.

Quantum leaps can also take place with human motivation. The base of the mountain represents having no desire to work toward a change of behavior, and the peak indicates a strong and ongoing drive to do all the things being a new person entails.

The traditional models of behavior change, as already discussed, involve climbing the mountain one step at a time. But a quantum leap takes a person's motivation right to the top. You are facing a mountain. You stand at the bottom. Peak motivation—your ultimate ability to do the work with inspired vigor—resides at the top. You can climb to that peak one step at a time (where there is risk of slipping and sliding back to the bottom anywhere along the route, but especially at the beginning), or you can step inside a *Star Trek*–style transporter device and materialize at the summit.

If you can locate such a transporter and figure out how to make it work, is it not worth giving it a shot if it means you get to bypass all those steps?

This does not mean the traditional model of slow-and-steady behavior change isn't sometimes worthwhile. This isn't one of those books filled with the Truth that "they" don't want you to know about. The reality is that millions *have* changed their lives via psychological baby steps, whereas many others achieve sudden change. And some people have experienced both types.

My friend Paul Ingraham, a health writer in Vancouver, has gone through three major behavioral changes in his life. Two of them were in the traditional linear fashion he called "forced marches across a tipping point; one desperate, determined step at a time." The other was via epiphany, which he described as "Way easier, completely irresistible. To have it was to change, no work required. Just *Poof!* I'm different now."

"Forced marches across a tipping point." This is an apt description for what most cognitive-behavior-change models are built around. But it doesn't always work that way.

I do not wish to dismiss decades of work by respected psychologists in the baby-steps approach to change, because it's a valuable tool that can be used to lead to epiphany. As I mentioned previously, look at the case of Lesley the fencer. She forced herself to struggle along for a couple of months, then came the *poof* Paul referred to. Same with my own physical transformation; I did not enjoy the first two months of battling to adopt an exercise regimen.

I struggled to develop the habit, and I almost quit. But when a staff member at the gym asked me if I'd had a good workout, and I realized that it *had* been pretty good, I had another epiphany: it was starting to *not suck*. And if it could not suck, then one day it could be enjoyable. In that moment, I promised myself I would keep exercising until I died. I met the *poof* partway, and over the next nine months, I lost fifty pounds of fat and gained twenty pounds of muscle. I've become a lifelong exerciser, going so far as to qualify for the Boston Marathon after seeing the horrific bombing in 2013, so I could run it the following year and be part of taking back the finish line from the terror of that day.

Time for another task.

Start thinking about what baby steps you can engage in to meet the *poof* partway. What is your desired outcome in terms of ultimate motivation? What is the peak of inspired Mount Everest in terms of what you could achieve for your life situation? Visualize that peak and what it would look like to be transported there, bypassing all intervening steps.

Now imagine the transporter device is broken and you need to hike a step at a time. Maybe not all the steps, but at least some. You can't stand around and wait for someone to fix the transporter. You need to start climbing.

What does the hike look like?

What is the first step?

Visualize your primary wish of this new person you'd like to be, whether it involves changes in activity level, diet, attitude, career, budgeting, education, a combination of any of these things, or some other things. Now forget that the transporter device exists.

What is the logical slow-and-steady path to achieve the goal? What is the first baby step? What is the second? The third? Start to map it out.

Create the beginnings of a plan to just get started. It's okay to seek help from a professional or otherwise knowledgeable person in formulating this plan.

Because the reality is, you may need to walk that path for a time. You may need to hike a while. But if you're attuned to the possibility of epiphany on that journey of many baby steps, the transporter may one day pick you up and materialize you at the peak. Or not quite at the peak, but a lot closer to the top, at least.

Sometimes the process is passive. It's something that happens to you, arriving unbidden. Other times, you must act.

Lace up those boots, because the *poof* is worth climbing toward.

The sudden-leap formula, which Ingraham described both as "way easier" and "completely irresistible," warrants further investigation so you can understand *why* it's worth the striving. Forced marches of motivation have a high failure rate, with not many people achieving lasting behavior change via such methods. This raises the question: What is the success rate of the quantum leap?

To uncover that, it is first important to gain deeper understanding of the mechanics of quantum change.

A Void in Need of Filling

"It's like a switch has been thrown and you've gone from where you used to be to somewhere else, and the intervening steps didn't occur," Rob Sawyer said. "That's a quantum change."

Sawyer's own change causing dramatic weight loss was quantum in nature. He spoke of twenty years at his sedentary job of being a writer leading to gaining significant weight, but he stayed affixed to that office chair because he had a mission.

"It was only when I won the Hugo Award for best novel [for *Hominids*] in 2003 when I had a void in my ambition that needed to be filled," he said. It was the top professional achievement he could attain in his field. Afterward, this other goal of losing weight that had been hovering in the background went through a quantum change. A return to discussing electrons explains how it happened.

"The lowest level of an atom holds two electrons, and the next highest level can hold eight," Sawyer said, explaining that you cannot push one of those lower-level electrons up to a higher state if all of those spots are occupied. But if one spot is vacated, there is an opportunity for a lower-level electron to complete a quantum leap to that higher level. It is promoted instantaneously. This is what happened for Sawyer. When he achieved ultimate career success, space was made for something else to become a top priority.

"It's no coincidence the year after winning the Hugo I lost a third of my body weight," Sawyer said. And true to the descriptions of it being a digital process and not analog, this or that, on or off, Rob was committed. "There was no wavering," he said. "It was going to happen."

Sawyer has kept the weight off more than a decade.

Make Room for Change

I have a big task for you now. So big, in fact, it needs its own header and section.

Reflect on what Sawyer said about winning the Hugo. Recall the description of how an electron at a higher level must vacate the premises prior to a lower-level electron being able to make that quantum leap to the higher energy level.

This is all about achieving a higher energy level.

And if your higher level is full, something needs to vacate it and make room for your inspiration to be instantaneously promoted, the way Rob's desire to lose weight was.

It's a fancy way of describing prioritization.

If your highest energy level is maxed out with "life stuff," you must reevaluate that stuff, because something needs to be deprioritized, perhaps even eliminated.

What takes up a lot of your energy?

Some things are critical. There are aspects of work and family that are challenging to deprioritize, but everyone wastes time, even those who think they don't. You say you need your downtime to watch TV or surf the net, but how much time? A 2016 Nielsen report determined that the average adult American spends over 4.5 hours each day watching TV shows and movies. This doesn't even consider surfing on your laptop or phone. Surely there is room to make room.

MAKE IT HAPPEN!

I have a few of these special exercises in the book. Call them "Act Now!" on steroids. I save them to call attention to more critical tasks. This one qualifies, because if a quantum leap of motivation is going to take place, your highest energy level needs an open slot. This is the detailed analysis, rather than sudden insight, for which writing things down may help. Examine your schedule and where your focus lies. Make a list of the stuff you do that sucks up a lot of energy and time. Consider where room can be made. You *need* this hole, this vacated spot, because then there will be a yearning to fill it. Give this task of making room the extra attention it deserves.

What may happen as a result of completing this first "Make It Happen!" exercise is that, through careful analysis, you determine, "Of course staring at a screen sucks up a lot of my time, so I'll just cut way back on that." But you don't. You keep staring, because it's paying off for you in some way.

But now you know this is part of the solution, and it sticks and gets unconsciously turned over, and then perhaps the epiphany comes through that uncovers *why* you have that behavior, how meaningless it is to continue the way you do, and how much more meaningful it would be to your life to spend that time on a passionate pursuit.

One day, you could be watching *The Big Bang Theory* and say, "Wow, this show has strapped a couple of hydrodynamic boards to its feet and achieved altitude overtop a carnivorous fish," and you start walking each evening instead.

The Ground Shifts

"This is about exponential change."

Ken Resnicow is a professor of health behavior at the University of Michigan and has published several papers on the phenomenon of quantum behavior change. He explained how the stages of change—the trans-theoretical model discussed in chapter 1—"is a very linear progression that is also quite proportional. They even talk about standard deviations of change." This means studies of TTM show groups of people based along a bell curve changing a specific amount at a specific rate.

Conversely, Rob Sawyer explained that quantum leaps of change are not linear, not proportional, and not in stages. "Exponential" means going from baby steps to Olympic-caliber long jump in a single stride.

"Using their terms [from Prochaska's TTM]," Resnicow said, "one can jump from precontemplator into action at a moment's notice." And this is not just action but *dedicated* action, aka "maintenance." In TTM, the "action" stage is tenuous. One is struggling to adopt the new behavior to achieve maintenance. But with a powerful epiphany there is no struggle; it is not a half-assed adoption. It's full-assed.

Lee Holland did not slowly slide over into laborious action because of her epiphany. Rather, she became dedicated to taking "action" regarding her career and into "maintenance" in an instant after the realization in the parking lot that she was destined to do much more with her life.

"Epiphany can be primed for," Resnicow said. "The raw materials for the perfect storm are something that can be provided." Priming can give people the information and skills that make it happen.

"Don't pressure yourself worrying that your light bulb hasn't gone off yet," Resnicow said. Doing so creates a state of anxiety. As we'll examine further, it's positive mood states that set the stage for sudden insight. Besides, "Sometimes things have to marinate for a while before epiphany happens."

It's a struggle to escape struggle.

Post-epiphany, the changes in behavior won't feel like work. It doesn't mean you don't have work to do first. I'm going to kick your ass a bit in coming chapters, and then, suddenly, perhaps . . .

"It isn't about struggling," said Professor Miller, who has been treating addictions for forty years. "With overcoming addiction, some people are often white-knuckle holding on to not go back to their previous situation." But he explained it is different for others, the ones who experience an epiphany, because they suddenly realize they've had enough.

"The typical epiphanies are, 'Oh, shit! I don't want to be this person anymore!'" said Resnicow. "If you're religious, it can be, 'This is not what God put me on Earth for.' It's an overwhelming sense the ground has shifted beneath you." Resnicow explained quantum change as a tectonic-plate movement in how you view your identity and your behavior, and how the two no longer are compatible.

An example of how well sudden change in behavior works comes from a 2009 study of seventeen hundred smokers and ex-smokers published in *Nicotine & Tobacco Research*. The authors found that those who spontaneously quit smoking are almost twice as likely to still not be smoking after six months than those who chose a carefully planned quitting attempt. It's also interesting that spontaneous quitters were less reliant upon pharmacotherapy to quit. They didn't need that nicotine patch. They were just done.

My best friend Craig woke up one day and promptly decided to quit when he realized how much money he'd wasted over the years. This cessation of smelling like an ashtray was done much to my and my wife's approval. After more than a quarter century, he's never wavered.

Battling addiction or weight or finding purpose are not the only things a quantum leap can assist with. A 2005 study published in *Behaviour Research and Therapy* looked at "sudden gains" in cognitive-behavioral treatment for depression. The research found not only did 42 percent of patients experience a great leap of improvement in a short time, but those who did were more likely to sustain such gains *and* had a higher rate of recovery.

I want to repeat something regarding epiphanies: It's not calculated. Professor Resnicow refers to it as a "metacognitive event." This means the solution to the problem often arrives while you're *not actively trying to solve the problem.*

For now, this is not helpful for those looking to achieve epiphany in order to change their lives. But I did the research and created a guaranteed* method for making it happen.

*JK. Not a guarantee.

Unlimited Drive

Until recently, the phenomenon of quantum change bestowing unlimited drive didn't mesh with research into "ego depletion," in which willpower is considered limited. Regular exertions of will to complete tasks or resist certain foods were thought to fatigue the mind; people run out of mental energy to adhere to their new lifestyle.

Imagine a bowl of radishes sits in front of you. How hard is it to resist eating them? How much *brainpower* does it require to not indulge? Cue people saying, "But I love radishes!" Yeah, whatever. Not the point, because most people don't love them.

Now imagine that same bowl filled with chocolate.

In 1998, a study of sixty-seven people was published in the *Journal of Personality and Social Psychology* describing an individual's willpower as a "limited resource" that is drained throughout the day each time it is utilized. Researchers took hungry people and told them they were to participate in a study about taste preferences. Faced with two food choices, chocolate treats or radishes, one group was told they had to "resist" the radishes and could only consume the chocolate, whereas the other group had the much more challenging task of not eating the treats that were right before them in favor of the radishes. Afterward, study participants were asked to work on an unsolvable puzzle.

They should have titled the study "Sometimes Scientists Are Dicks."

Those asked to abstain from chocolate gave up on the puzzle faster than those who ate chocolate but no radishes. Researchers concluded the stress of resisting chocolate drained the participants' willpower, causing them to give up on the puzzle sooner. Like when you have a shit day at work and are more likely to hit the liquor store on the way home instead of the gym.

This willpower study received international attention and launched further research into ego depletion, leading scientists to recommend that people interested in behavior change not alter too many things at once or too drastically, else they risk depleting their willpower and sabotaging their efforts. Quitting smoking and drinking, switching to healthier eating, and adopting an exercise regimen all at once was a recipe for failure, whereas making small, incremental steps toward adopting new habits was encouraged.

But these recommendations, it turns out, were based on bad assumptions.

Researchers from Curtin University in Australia conducted a meta-analysis of two dozen studies of ego depletion involving over two thousand subjects. Published in 2016 in *Perspectives on Psychological Science,* the study found no evidence of ego depletion; the entire concept was deemed faulty. I spoke with Professor Michael Inzlicht, whom you'll recall from the previous chapter, and who has long been a critic of the concept of ego depletion, to learn more about why we shouldn't consider willpower as a tank that can be emptied.

"There are many potential reasons why self-control might wane over time," Inzlicht said. He dismissed the idea of will as a resource, countering that people's preferences change over time. And in the case of epiphany, "over time" can mean the space of a few seconds. A 2007 study published in *Counselling & Psychotherapy Research* examined how insight can act as a shortcut to personal growth. Many interview subjects for the study described the specific moment their lives transformed; it wasn't a glacial process, but rather instantaneous.

How did ego depletion gain such traction? It turns out that the problem lay with how studies prior to the twenty-first century were designed. When more modern statistical analysis is used, Inzlicht explained, the effect of ego depletion disappears. "At the very best, it's a small effect."

There has been a revolution in how research is conducted, and psychology is in the middle of it. Numerous old findings are turning out to not be as robust as once thought. Professor Inzlicht explained it wasn't specific to the radish-vs.-chocolate study, but to all studies of the era. "Everyone was doing it," he said.

Doing what? Hunting for a significant effect via "P-hacking." The "P" stands for "probability"; it involves dredging through the collected data to uncover a pattern that can be presented as statistically significant.

On the same day as my conversation with Inzlicht, there was serendipitously a feature published in *The New York Times* discussing this exact phenomenon in reference to Harvard social psychologist Amy Cuddy. She used the methods of the day to create an influential study on "power poses"—how certain standing and sitting positions influence people's feeling of power. Publication launched her career to new heights, but her failure to replicate her findings using new methods of analysis brought out the critics. Fellow academics "savaged" her work and career. Power posing was referred to as "inconsequential" for helping people "do better in life."

Add "publication bias" to this, which Inzlicht explained this way: "What if I told you twenty studies were run and only the three with significant findings were published?" If no effect is shown, they don't get published. "They are hidden in the proverbial file drawer."

Inzlicht says willpower isn't a tank but has more to do with desire and drive. "Sometimes those desires change gradually; others, they turn on a dime."

The dime-turning of desire—that's what a sudden identity-value shift does. What once was difficult is now easy or even effortless. It's not because willpower became abundant; it's because values changed. "It calls for a radical shift in how we perceive self-control," Inzlicht said.

The 2016 study of the identity-value model of self-control mentioned in the previous chapter examined a number of more recent studies finding that what we imagine as ego depletion could be quickly eliminated via things such as pondering positive outcomes, taking a break to watch TV, experiencing a positive mood change, meditating, or even praying.

And a 2017 study of 258 people by researchers at the University of Zurich put another nail in the coffin. It found that merely discussing the idea of ego depletion creates a self-fulfilling prophecy, because people are prone to suggestibility. In one study, participants who were told that a mentally challenging task would lead to ego depletion became fatigued afterward. Conversely, those who were told the same challenging task would energize them for subsequent tasks were indeed energized.

Can you pump up your willpower like a muscle? Can you *train* it to be stronger? The research isn't promising. A 2016 meta-analysis published in *Health Psychology Review* examined training people to resist temptations of things such as alcohol and snack food, and found it only worked in the short term. More disconcerting is a study published the same year in the *Journal of Experimental Psychology* that put 174 participants through six weeks of self-control training. The authors stated their study "rectified several methodological problems with previous studies and observed that self-control training did not improve self-control."

What is the secret of those who are successful at self-control?

Inzlicht coauthored a 2017 study published in *Social Psychological and Personality Science* that examined "effortful self-control" in the face of temptation. He told me of how the researchers asked people about short-term goals, then followed up three months later to ascertain their success. "The biggest contributor to meeting or showing progress toward their goals was whether they encountered temptation." If they experienced a desire that conflicted with their goals (cake vs. weight loss, Facebook vs. studying), effortful resisting of the desire *made no difference*. The ones who made progress were those who *avoided being tempted in the first place*.

A key aspect of avoiding temptation? Don't feel it any longer. That comes via the shift in identity and values. If your new passion overrides distractions, they don't distract you.

Sometimes it doesn't even require an epiphany to make this shift, but a simple reframing of the self for generating situation-specific self-control. A 2012 study published in the *Journal of Consumer Research* examined "empowered refusal" of temptation and discovered that those who used "I don't" language (as in "I don't eat chocolate cake") were almost twice as successful at resisting temptation than those who used "I can't" language. This ties back to identity and how we view ourselves. Those who shift their identity and values achieve a potentially limitless source of drive to pursue the behaviors aligning with those values and that identity.

What about those who don't shift identities but power through with effortful exertion of self-control because they have "grit"? Such people exist, but grittiness may not be good for them. A 2015 study of 292 African

American teenagers from disadvantaged backgrounds published in *Psychological and Cognitive Sciences* discovered that those who were better at using self-control and had "the ability to resist temptations that interfere with long-term aspirations" suffered negative health consequences, such as increased stress responses and even premature aging of immune cells. This is in line with previous studies showing that while such enforced self-control improves psychosocial outcomes, it worsens cardiometabolic health. It's far better, and easier, to *remove* feelings of temptation—whatever they may be—than to engage in continual resistance.

Earlier, we analyzed quantum leaps, and it is worth noting that "quantum" derives from the word "quantity"; in physics, quanta refers to a unit of energy. A quantum leap, in turn, describes a sudden movement from one *energy level* to another. A quantum leap of motivation, therefore, is about instantaneously achieving an increase in energy to pursue change because who you are and what your values are have changed.

Those who believe they have unlimited mental energy to pursue a new path pursue it. Although not the best analogy from a scientific perspective, emotionally I am reminded of one of the final scenes from *Indiana Jones and the Last Crusade*. Indy's father, played by Sean Connery, has been shot and lies dying. His only hope resides in a miracle: the healing power of the Holy Grail. To save his father, Indy is told, "It's time to ask yourself what you believe."

To experience an identity-altering moment that makes major life change sustainable, it is important to believe such events do not *just happen* but *can* happen to you. That's why I'm going deep into the science. I'm not asking you to take it on faith, but to examine the evidence and come to your own conclusions.

So, Indy, what *do* you believe?

Understanding When Epiphany Strikes

A question worth pondering is: "How does a person *know* when they've experienced a life-changing epiphany?" It appears the answer is: *They just know.* Nevertheless, William Miller provided clarification of the characteristics of quantum change in a 2004 paper published in the *Journal of Clinical Psychology*:

These characteristics include:

- Distinctiveness: People knew this was an extraordinary event.
- Surprise: It was sudden and unexpected.
- Benevolence: It came with a positive sense of self and safety.
- Permanence: The change stuck.

Epiphany can strike at any time. Professor Miller spoke of one man who had his epiphany while walking across his living room; another recipient was a woman who was cleaning the toilet.

I had an epiphany while cleaning the toilet. Suddenly, I was struck with an overwhelming passion for teaching a little boy how to aim.

Recall the emotion-driven animal. When a quantum-leaping elephant crashes down upon an epiphany landing pad, it's going to make an impression, but in *Quantum Change* Miller explains there is a "bimodal distribution" of the experience, with "insightful" epiphanies at one end of the continuum and "mystical" at the other.

The Insightful Epiphany

The insightful epiphany is analogous to looking at Gestalt figures. These are images, usually in black-and-white, that can be seen two different ways to reveal two different things.

"It's like the drawing of a woman where if you look at it one way, you see a young woman," Miller said, "but if you look at it another way, you see an old woman." Once you've seen the old woman, you can't *unsee* it. (That drawing is at the beginning of this book, opposite the title page.)

This particular illusion first dates back to an 1888 German postcard and has since become known as the "Boring figure," named after psychologist Edwin Boring, who wrote a paper about it in 1930. It became a key example among Gestalt figures. Gestalt is a form of psychology that involves finding meaningful perceptions in a chaotic world. *Gestalt* is a German word that means "shape" or "form" and, in essence, refers to how the whole is greater than the sum of its parts.

Massive and sudden insight into one's life involves a reorganization of information in the brain. The various "parts" of data, knowledge, and experience *gel* in a profound way so the new whole is unique, profound, enlightening, and inspiring.

With Lee Holland, she had a sudden insight that she had the ability to help people in a way she never could in her present job. My first big one also qualifies as the insightful type of epiphany.

In *The Eureka Factor,* Kounios and Beeman refer to such sudden insight as "quantum leaps of thought, creative breakthroughs that power our lives." They added, "They can and do change lives."

The Mystical Experience

"These are profoundly spiritual experiences," William Miller said of mystical epiphanies. He also explained that this type of experience has been well described for centuries, with religious texts being one example of where they are often recorded. A mystical experience typically starts abruptly, and the person understands *something unusual* is happening to them. That's what happened in this next story you're about to read. Miller said, "It is common to feel a sense of unity with all of creation or humanity."

What is interesting is that Miller said most of the people they talked to who had this kind of experience weren't often religious.

Do you, dear reader, need to be concerned over whether an epiphany is mystical or insightful, or somewhere on the continuum in between? I'd say no. You don't need to label it.

You just need to try to experience it.

Dying for Change

Except I don't advise trying to experience this, because "this" is where "how to" goes out the window.

The world doesn't need another reboot of the *Flatliners* movie as a way to induce a mystical epiphany. There's a reason the 2017 version only got a 5 percent score on Rotten Tomatoes. Dying on purpose to see what's on the other side is a *bad idea*.

Josie Thomson's story isn't from a movie. She had a mystical life-changing moment from a near-death experience that *is* worth telling. It was 1991, and the then twenty-four-year-old lived in Melbourne, Australia. She was newly married, a practicing Catholic from a large Italian family. She didn't smoke or drink, she exercised regularly, and she had a promising career with a multi-national corporation.

Despite being young and taking good care of herself, Josie had a ticking time bomb inside her. A lump in her throat that wouldn't go away was the harbinger of change.

An ultrasound revealed it to be a thyroid tumor that was at first thought to be minor. She was told she'd only need to spend twenty-four hours in the hospital, but after it was excised, she and her husband were kept waiting for several hours. Finally, the doctor came in, his eyes red, and said, "I don't know how to tell you this. It's stage three malignant cancer." Another, much more invasive procedure on her neck area was needed.

"My husband fell apart," Josie said. "I remembered looking at him and thinking, *Imagine what I feel like!*" She needed him to be strong for her, but he wasn't. He couldn't cope with the situation. Her second surgery was scheduled for the next morning, and when her then husband left the hospital that evening he gave her a telling look. "There were no words exchanged," she said. "I just knew he would never come back, and he never did."

The worst was yet to come. The surgery devastated Josie's body; she lost a lot of blood, and her vital signs crashed, putting her in the intensive-care unit. She was so weak that on the second day after surgery, her heart stopped beating: flatline.

"Then the most curious thing occurred," Josie told me. "All of a sudden, part of me was on the ceiling, looking down at my physical body. There was no emotion. Just pure serenity. I was aware it was my body below me on the bed, and I saw doctors and nurses frantically attending me, but I felt so peaceful." Then, she said, she heard a stern male voice command her: "It's not your time yet." And she felt catapulted back into her body.

Belief in such out-of-body experiences is a matter of individual faith. What is undeniable is that whatever it was that happened to Josie Thomson in that hospital room changed the path of her life.

"I remember it all so clearly, as if it happened yesterday. It was the beginning of my spiritual journey in earnest. Everything I had been taught to blindly believe in was now up for negotiation." She spoke with the archbishop about her experience and didn't get satisfactory answers. "I realized Catholicism was not the path for me. I wound up exploring a whole range of other things." Because of her experience, Josie says she no longer fears death. Now remarried with two children that she was told she'd likely never be able to have, her spirituality aligns more with Hinduism and Buddhism. She meditates every day and feels deeply connected to the world.

Her spirituality was not the only thing that changed. "Being the eldest daughter of an Italian family, my middle names were 'duty' and 'obligation,'" she said, only partially joking. The near-death experience taught her to say no to people. "That was the moment I decided to live life on my own terms."

Shortly after leaving the hospital, the company she worked for offered her a job in Brisbane, over a thousand miles from home. Despite her family's protestations and not having fully recovered from surgery, she took it.

The experience taught Josie to forge her own path. "Before, I was this compliant and obedient good girl, always trying to please and appease and be accepted. But all the while I was rejecting my true self and never able to do what was right for me."

In 2001, Josie made a career change to be an executive coach and is now a sought-after and award-winning public speaker. She said her life is amazing, and upon waking each day she gives thanks for being alive.

"It was when my throat was cut open that I found my voice," she said.

Quantum Stickiness

Failure is common in life-change endeavors. Chances are, you have tried and failed to go through a significant altering of behavior at least once.

For few, it seems, *dramatic* behavior change is a linear process. The ones who went through a massive shift had a holy-shit life-changing moment.

There is no shortage of personal stories describing such an event. Alas, the plural of "anecdote" is not "data." Fortunately, the available scientific evidence legitimizes such anecdotes of sudden and lasting change.

The research mentioned earlier regarding depression showed those who made something akin to a quantum change were more likely to sustain their improvements than those who took a more linear path. There are also the studies about the smokers being much more successful when they'd suddenly quit than those who'd had a plan. Also interesting is the ten-year follow-up with the subjects interviewed for William Miller's book about quantum change.

Janet C'de Baca, who was a clinical psychologist in Albuquerque and Professor Miller's coauthor on the book, tracked down thirty of the fifty-five people interviewed for *Quantum Change.* Publishing her results in 2004 in the *Journal of Clinical Psychology,* she found that "These dramatic changes have continued, and none described a return to old ways of being."

Embrace Chaos

You know that quote about the definition of insanity often attributed to Albert Einstein? The one that says it's "doing the same thing over and over again and expecting a different result"?

It likely wasn't Einstein who came up with it, as no reliable evidence has been supplied to show him as the originator. What's more, Alice Calaprice, editor of *The Ultimate Quotable Einstein,* puts the quote in the "Misattributed to Einstein" section at the end of the book. Instead, the quote appears to have been adapted from a 1981 Narcotics Anonymous pamphlet, which states, "Insanity is repeating the same mistakes and expecting different results." And yet most people believe it was Einstein. I guess there really is a sucker born every minute. By the way, P. T. Barnum never actually said that.

I'll stop now.

Embracing chaos to achieve epiphany means ceasing the same-old. If you desire a quantum change in your motivation to succeed at something, you're going to have to try some new and potentially frightening things.

When William Miller began his research into quantum change, the goal was to determine if it was even a legitimate experience. His opinion? "Having done the study, I have no question that it is a real phenomenon." As a reminder, Miller explained it's not even that uncommon, with as many as one-third of people experiencing such an event during their lives.

What if we can boost that figure?

Think about it. A third are experiencing epiphany, mostly coming out of nowhere. Now that we're studying it in depth and analyzing the triggers and *pushing* you to make it happen, perhaps the odds climb to half, even higher.

Maybe, if you understand the science, if you work the plan, if you take these tasks to heart, your odds of making this happen are better than half. You work until you're stuck. Then you divert. Then **Poof*!*

You are different. What you experienced is not a change in motivation, it's a change in you.

How big is the payout?

Such an endeavor is not "win big or don't win at all." Yes, you can go from unlit match to a raging bonfire of inspiration, but being presented with a toasty campfire is still good. It's less like roulette and more like a slot machine. Sometimes the sudden gains are all three bars; other times, it's three cherries. As I mentioned, the course correction of the new path can be big or . . . less big.

When your brain lights up, and you feel the power of inspiration upon you, the sense of rightness is reminiscent of Roger Daltrey from The Who singing "Won't Get Fooled Again." You feel a sudden change, and it affirms your new purpose with a "Yeah!" like the one the vocalist lets loose four and a half minutes into the song. But that's the "less big," toasty campfire version. The raging bonfire proclamation is a few minutes later, toward the end of the 1971 hit. Like what happened to so many of the people I spoke with for this book, the feeling of rightness is akin to one of the greatest voices in the history of rock and roll erupting with a volcanic "*YEEE-AAAAHHHHH!!!*"

Except, you know, in your mind.

Want that feeling? Again, for the magic to work, Indy, it helps if you believe.

Except it's not magic, it's psychology. The human brain is extraordinarily complex, and our understanding of it is far from complete. We do know belief is a powerful motivator, so if you can accept the scientific validity, if you can imagine that your life may turn on a dime in a moment, the odds increase.

But you're not waiting for the random playing of that song. Rather than trust fate, you're digging through your pocket for quarters. You're getting out of a chair and ambling toward the jukebox. You flip through selections and find the right one. You put in your money, make your selection, and you wait.

And maybe the power goes out and nothing happens. But maybe . . . maybe Roger's voice is crisp and clear and explodes into your mind, and you realize with a "Holy freaking shit!" what I'm talking about. This new boss of your life, this new passion, will be nothing like the old boss.

The phenomenon of a life-changing moment, from a psychological research perspective, is in its infancy. But Ken Resnicow doesn't see that linear and quantum models of behavior change need be at odds. In 2008, he had an article published in the *American Journal of Public Health* that looked at how we normally see behavior change—as a rational, reductionist model that is proportional (small inputs = small outputs)—and how real life is often a chaotic process that is unpredictable. In the article, Resnicow examined how life transformation can arrive beyond cognition, and how it is necessary for the psychological community to take a more serious look at integrating a "complex systems" approach to public health with the current, more linear model of behavior change.

Can a person stack the deck? Can they *make* epiphany happen? Can rational and chaotic processes work in concert to change one's life for the better?

Professor Resnicow is adamant they can. So is Professor Beeman, who we'll be learning much more from regarding the neuroscience of epiphany in chapter 4. I'm convinced as well, because not only did I make it happen for myself, I've helped make it happen for others.

Let's try another experiment. It's time to change the initial conditions, to introduce some chaos and see which way the droplet rolls.

To start, imagine a time when you were successful at change; those self-efficacy performance accomplishments discussed earlier. Imagine a time when you needed to adopt that Nike slogan and "Just do it." Try to recall, *how* did you "just do" that? Where did the motivation come from? Make some mental notes about what you were feeling. Was there something unique about the experience?

Because maybe we don't need to reinvent the wheel. Maybe you already have the skills of rapid and massive change because you've done it before but forgot. Daydream a little. Take a long, insightful look back, and ponder. . . .

Nothing yet? Dig a little deeper. Go back a little farther. Maybe there is something that doesn't seem significant now, but at the time was important. You may have been a child. Perhaps it involved standing up to a bully or finding the courage to do something you were terrified of. Were you sweating bullets going into that job interview but pulled yourself together and crushed it? Can you recall how you approached the problem? Was there some secret to your success in overcoming?

Take your time. Think a while. It's okay if, after a while, you say, "I got nothin'." It's all part of getting stuck before the distraction that permits insight to arrive, seemingly unbidden.

But the insight was totally bidden. This whole book is about extending epiphany an invitation, hoping it will show up at some random point and get the party started.

You don't always have to dwell on the problem, but rather do some stuff while the problem resides adjacent and hope the solution will coalesce and perhaps arrive via your unconscious.

Maybe you need to go outside.

"We've known for a long time that writers get benefit from being active out in nature," Ruth Ann Atchley, a psychology professor at the University of Kansas, told me. "The environment makes a big difference." Atchley, who has a special interest in this subject and has published research about improving creative reasoning in natural settings, explained that it's a synergistic effect of not only engaging physical activity but doing it outside, away from modern technological distractions.

Much of what we're trying to do in this book is linked to creative thought; creativity isn't limited to your ability to paint or compose music.

"Aerobic exercise is very beneficial for thinking and cognition," she said. It enhances the function of the prefrontal cortex, which is important for creativity and moving attention from task to task.

But could walking on a treadmill in your basement get the same result? Answer: no. It is beneficial to get away from the technology-rich environment, Atchley explained. Reading email and checking your phone takes you off task and inhibits creativity for as long as five minutes each time, she said, so leave the phone at home.

The natural environment has a characteristic some call "soft fascination." This means the environmental stimuli are emotionally positive, and positivity is integral to triggering sudden insight (details in chapter 4). "The natural environment has the ability to seduce and *attract* your attention system rather than *demand* it," she said. Emails, ringing phones, and Facebook notifications are demanding of your attention, but nature is cool with you just hanging out with her. You know, soaking things in. Gently.

But for enhancing creative thinking, the type of exercise matters. The level of arousal needs to be low.

Professor Atchley likes to snowshoe and downhill-ski, and she explained, "The level of arousal in snowshoeing is not very stimulating, so it's good for enhancing creative thinking. But the skiing creates a heightened state of arousal. It requires more attention."

I am also a skier, and I know my brain is often focused on things such as: *Turn. Turn again. Moguls! Watch out for that tree. Squirrel!*

Effort matters as well. As the exercise becomes more demanding, these creative cognitive benefits of being in a natural environment diminish. I'm more creative while cycling at a moderate intensity, but during a hard run my brain gets distracted with thoughts of *Gasp! I hate this hill. My heart hurts.*

The lesson is, go outside, keep the arousal of the activity low and the intensity moderate.

How large is the effect?

Atchley and her team use word problems—called a Remote Associates Test, something we'll examine in detail later—and found exercising in nature garnered a 50 percent increase in creative thinking over being sedentary indoors, a substantial improvement indeed.

There will be many other detailed suggestions to come, but for now, after you ponder to the point you can't ponder anymore and you get stuck, go outside and get lost in thought.

And the ground may shift. If you're in Los Angeles or San Francisco and feel the earth move, look around and see if other people are freaking out. If not, it was an epiphany.

Don't discount any weird way to experience that which is new or exotic.

Embrace chaos. Embrace opportunity. Embrace change.

Challenge your mind to seek out new experiences and new ways of thinking.

And stay attuned throughout the process. As I wrote earlier: *Seek* the magic moment, and if something tickles, don't push it down, float it up. Turn it over. See if it can grow from "maybe something" into "definitely a thing."

Do all this, because when initial conditions are changed, the brain begins to fire in unique ways, increasing the possibility that *your solution* will suddenly appear. Sometimes the sword needs to already be gripped to awaken the desire to become a master of the blade.

With this discussion of quantum leaps of motivation, we've gone far beyond the common models of cognitive behavior change, and we're not stopping here. In the ensuing chapters, we'll take a broader look at human behavior and how both rational and irrational thinking, as well as simple vs. complex decision-making processes, affect what we do and how we find purpose.

Act Now!

- Start planning the baby steps you would need to take to "meet the *poof* partway." Using the regular, gradual approach to behavior change, imagine what it would take for that first step, the second, and so on.
- Make room for change. Look at what occupies your "highest energy level," and find things that can be deprioritized or even eliminated so your new quest has room for being promoted. Understand you may need to dig deep to first understand why you spend time on a wasteful activity before discarding it.
- Don't worry that your light bulb hasn't gone off yet, because it doesn't happen while you're thinking about it.
- Stop viewing willpower as a limited resource, and instead seek a shift in identity and values that makes the new, desired behaviors mandatory.
- Embrace new and "chaotic" ways of thinking. Try meditating or getting out in nature or even prayer. Realize you need to break out of the same old routine; you need to try not just doing new things, but *thinking* new things.
- Spend some time outside as a diversion from planning and pondering. Keep the arousal low (simple walking vs. a task requiring coordination) and the effort no more than moderate.
- And finally, unless you're the type who despises classic rock, pull out your phone and activate The Google. Type in "the who won't get fooled again" and have a listen. Feel free to plug in your headphones and give the volume a crank. The first "Yeah!" is at 4:28. Ponder the moderate, toasty campfire power of it. Keep listening. The next one has a slow build with that seventies "I was high on something when I wrote this"

endless synthesizer coupled with mad drumming going on and on, because back then radio stations were okay with playing songs eight and a half minutes long. It finally hits at 7:45, and it's awesome. That's your brain on bonfire. That's your kick-ass, life-will-never-be-the-same righteous realization. Commit to strive for it.

P.S. I saw The Who perform on their fiftieth-anniversary tour. They still got it.

Yeah.

3

YOU, PART 2:

FINDING PURPOSE VIA EPIPHANY

A ship in harbor is safe, but that is not what ships are built for.
—JOHN A. SHEDD

I am a horrible person.

Speaking of horrible people, Ayn Rand rejected altruism. Friedrich Nietzsche argued it's self-motivated. Psychologists and philosophers alike have analyzed the behavior, with some saying true altruism doesn't exist.

This is a tale for the "doesn't exist" because "self-motivated" column.

My son was soon leaving for the day's first-year engineering classes. I knew he would want food prior to going to school. "Would you like me to make you an omelet?" I asked.

"Yes, please."

I make omelets for him often. He likes my cooking, and there is a parental instinct to shove food in the face holes of our offspring. It initiates a dopamine cascade for having fulfilled one's genetic destiny, or some shit.

Anyway . . . me: horrible.

I made my son a nice ham-and-cheese omelet, just the way he likes it.

He ate it. He enjoyed it. He went to school.

What was in it for me?

There is something else in the fridge.

We have leftover butter chicken, rice, and naan from the local Indian restaurant. I knew if he relied on cooking for himself, he'd nuke the leftovers. Now he is gone, belly full of the tasty omelet I made him. And the leftovers are here. They are all mine.

I'm eating butter chicken as I write this. It's delicious. I feel like I earned it.

Does true altruism exist? Who cares? But realize you're not a bad person if your epiphany seems self-serving rather than prompts you to dedicate your life to saving the Australian drop bear from extinction. It's okay to choose the path best for *you*. Perhaps, as a bonus, you can find one that also helps others.

What is your purpose? Why are you here? What does the universe want of you?

I don't imagine the universe gives a flatulent gas giant if we live or die. I expect humanity is just some shit that happened. This doesn't mean I don't put high value on the power of having purpose in life.

Whatever you believe—if we are divinely created beings or semisentient stardust meat sacks—is fine by me. Perhaps we'll find out if the purpose we were inspired to live was "right" on the day we commence decomposition. In the meantime, the tools I prefer are science, logic, and a wee bit o' philosophy to help us along the way to figuring out You, Part 2.

Speaking of beliefs . . .

"You are stronger than you believe. You have greater powers than you know." That's from *Wonder Woman,* said by Antiope, played by Robin Wright, as she's teaching young Diana to kick the ass of whichever foe is stupid enough to get in her way. If you've seen the film and Antiope's death scene didn't wrench your guts, you are dead inside.

We all have reservoirs of strength and courage that can see us through challenges to achieve lofty goals, if you feel destined to achieve these goals, if you believe doing so is tied to your identity.

Identity, passion, and values can align in myriad ways. It may have to do with parenting, relationships, volunteering, physical accomplishment, career, or a combination. It may regard mood state. If you've lived the life of a cynic who always presumes the worst, that can change in an instant.

In *The Eureka Factor,* Kounios and Beeman explain that figuring out goals related to purpose in life are "too fuzzy and complicated for you to methodically evaluate all the possibilities." And so, this is an area where "insight shines."

Achieving insight is about gathering information, then letting the unconscious work on it.

Ancient Wisdom for the Modern Human

Why are you here? Let's ask some dead people.

Twentieth-century French philosopher Jean-Paul Sartre said it's for no particular reason. "Existence precedes essence," he famously said in Paris, just a few months after the end of the Second World War. Sartre proclaimed there is no God and therefore we are not created for a purpose. Whoa, sounds dark. Fear not, unbelievers in a higher power. Sartre relishes in the liberty such thinking entails. If nothing is fixed, we have the freedom to create purpose for ourselves.

But such freedom comes with responsibility, the greatest responsibility of all: If nothing is preordained, we are condemned to consider the impact of our choices upon all humankind. There is more to life than looking out for number one.

Or you may say to hell with that.

Albert Camus, another French philosopher of the same era as Sartre, wrote, "Life will be lived all the better if it has no meaning." It's worth noting he was living in Nazi-occupied France at the time; it may have affected his mood. He wasn't a complete downer, though. Camus added, "The struggle itself towards the heights is enough to fill a man's heart." I'm writing this in 2018; I prefer "human" over "man," but you get the idea. Speaking of 2018, Nazis are still bad. FYI.

Here's a tongue twister for you: *eudaimonia*.

It's ancient Greek, referring to "human flourishing." It was mostly an Aristotelian thing; he wrote about it in his *Nicomachean Ethics* in the fourth century BC. It's not just about living well but doing things well. You can have skills or virtues, but you also must act upon them. You can do this for the betterment of yourself, but it's even cooler if humanity also benefits. Sir Winston Churchill drove it home: "What is the use of living, if it be not to strive for noble causes and to make this muddled world a better place for those who will live in it after we are gone?"

That's flourishing.

William Du Bois, a political activist and the first African American to obtain a doctorate from Harvard, asserted the importance of belief for *eudaimonia* to be achieved: we need to "Believe in life!" We must imagine that progress and a fuller life are *possible*.

Believing is one thing; practicality still plays a role.

"I am myself and my circumstances." These are the words of Spanish philosopher José Ortega y Gasset, written in his 1914 book *Meditations on Quixote*. Our situation can be both oppressive and limiting. Our circumstances come not just from the physical world, but our own minds. Mental health, prejudices, and preconceptions all affect our ability to flourish. We can imagine new possibilities, but they will run into our present circumstances. And so he wrote, "Life is a series of collisions with the future."

That being written, Ortega believed that to live "like everyone else" was to lack personal vision or moral code. He wanted people to look at their lives with fresh eyes, engage creatively, and commit to formulating new possibilities, all while using reason to create that vital energy that spurs us forward.

That seems like a good dead-guy analysis to end the philosophical section on.

Truth and Consequences

Choosing a new path has consequences. William James (also dead) is acknowledged as the Father of American Psychology. When it comes to *what* happened regarding a life-changing epiphany, he wrote in 1902, psychologists can provide a general description, but *how* or *why* such events come to be are less discernable.

Finding your truth via a holy-shit moment is not to be pursued lightly. Because consequences.

Consider what they might be. James was also considered the Father of

American Pragmatism. Don't let principles or belief systems steer you off a cliff. Consider the long-term destination of any new path.

As explained, the "fast" way of thinking, System 1 (elephant), constructs the story, and System 2 (rider) believes it. System 2 is the rational, slower part of the brain. If it throws up red flags, proceed with caution.

But sometimes we throw caution to the wind because we are compelled. Usually, according to the research of Professor William Miller and the numerous interviews I conducted for this book, such ambitious endeavors work out, even if at first it is a rough road. Chasing of lofty goals is not being cavalier, it's being determined and fearless.

In *Quantum Change,* Miller and C'de Baca outlined "five perspectives" on why a person has a life-changing epiphany. Sometimes it's a "breaking point": You just can't do you the same way any longer. The current path of your life becomes intolerable. This is covered further in chapter 5, where we examine hitting rock bottom. Another perspective is "personal maturation," except in a "spurt" as opposed to being gradual. A "sacred encounter," similar to what Josie Thomson experienced and which we examine further in chapter 6, is another. The one I want to focus on for finding purpose in life is "deep discrepancy." It's the proverbial wake-up call regarding your sense of self. You aren't at a breaking point, but something triggers a higher awareness that things aren't right. Then, shift happens.

Miller told me we tend to stay on a given path until something triggers us that change is needed.

Social psychologist Roy Baumeister wrote a chapter for a 1994 book about personality change referring to "the crystallization of discontent." He explained, prior to such crystallization, "a person may have many complaints and misgivings about some role, relationship, or involvement, but these remain separate from each other." When the "totality" of these negative features is achieved by creating "associative links," then "the subjective impact can be enormous." Baumeister refers to these as "focal incidents" that can "call attention to problems that have already existed."

Ken Resnicow cautions against making the focus negative. "When someone proclaims, 'Oh, shit! I'm a hypocrite.' Or, 'I'm a bad Christian!' they view it as 'I'm filthy. I must be purified.'" He asserted the need to view such crystallization as a more positive phenomenon. As mentioned, a positive mood is more likely to generate sudden insight. "You don't want a negative tone in your motivational thinking."

In relation to epiphany, Miller and C'de Baca examined Rokeach's "Model of Personality." It's reminiscent of *Shrek,* in which he says ogres are like onions. *Layers!*

The outer layer in Rokeach's model is superficial action and thoughts. Go down a level and the layer is beliefs, then attitudes, values, and, finally, the self. The authors explain that the more central the level at which someone changes, the more it will endure and the greater impact it will have.

Going to the gym is a superficial action requiring exertion of will. Conversely, having health be a core value removes the struggle to be active, can even make it enjoyable. It can do the same for quitting bad habits such as smoking or drinking.

Because you are so much more than your actions.

In her book *Mindfulness,* Ellen Langer—the first woman to ever become a tenured professor of psychology at Harvard—writes of how focusing on outcome narrows self-image. That's not good, because basing who you are, judging it on your past performance, is limiting and *inhibiting*.

A couple more dead philosophers, okay?

At his trial for being "a corruptor of the youth" and not believing in "the gods of the state," Plato wrote that Socrates proclaimed, "The life which is unexamined is not worth living." Søren Kierkegaard, a nineteenth-century Dane, explained that such self-analysis is how we understand despair. In so doing, people often wish to be other than who they are, to change the self. Yet that is problematic, because they're looking to become someone different, and there is no good outcome. If they fail at the attempt, they hate themselves for failing, and if they succeed, they abandon their true selves, which also leads to despair.

You must find the *true self.* All this stuff about identity shifts and becoming a different person in a moment is still in line with Kierkegaard's teachings; it's about accepting *who you really are*—the *best* version of it— and bringing it to the surface, letting it be in charge. Twentieth-century German psychoanalyst Karen Horney expanded upon this by comparing the "real self," which contains our authentic desires, with the "ideal self," which strives to fulfill all those "shoulds" that external forces impose and that can tyrannize one's life. If we ignore the real in favor of the ideal, and fail, this leads to development of the "despised self."

It's been a little while since I gave you a task. I've been saving it up. I am going to ask you a big question. Perhaps *the* big question:

Who are you?

Time for another one of those special exercises.

MAKE IT HAPPEN!

Ask, who is your real self? What are your values? What is *most important* to you? Have you even considered it? Are these values you hold outdated and in need of an upgrade? How do you feel about things like generosity, spirituality, or honesty? What value do you place on health, family, or love?

Also examine where there is discontent as it relates to your core values. As Resnicow warns, it's not good to dwell on the negative, but crystallization can lead to action, so don't discard the power of dissatisfaction with the path you're on.

Ask yourself: What values do I need to let reign in order to *flourish* as a human?

Examine your truth, but don't forget to consider the consequences of a shift in values. Store it away in the brain. Spin it around. Ponder, ruminate, and repeat. Get stuck, then get outside. Stay attuned for achieving a focal point. You know the drill.

Let's drive home this concept of letting inner values reign with a quick story from Professor Sherry Pagoto. She told me of a woman who was depressed, inactive, and had obesity. A core value for her was a love of animals. Upon examining this, she aligned her behavior with it and began volunteering at an animal shelter to walk dogs, and it clicked for her. She had an epiphany that this simple act was something with the power to change her life, and it did. "The person realizes, *I had no idea this would give me such a thrill!*" Pagoto said. "Then they can't stop doing it." They can't stop, because the inner-layer value drives the outer-layer behavior.

Lesson: Dogs = good.

Behaving Economically

Decisions, decisions. Life change comes with risk.

In 1979, Daniel Kahneman and his partner Amos Tversky published a landmark study with the title "Prospect Theory: An Analysis of Decision Under Risk." The study became a foundation of behavioral economics and led to Kahneman winning the Nobel Memorial Prize in Economic Sciences in 2002 (despite being a psychologist who never studied economics).

Simply put, the theory asserts that people make decisions based more upon *potential value* of losses and gains rather than on actual outcome. And they assess potential value using mental shortcuts that give weight to certain aspects of a problem while ignoring others. These are intuitive judgments.

So what? It gives us a bit of insight into how our minds work and how fear or discontent can lead to sudden change.

A 2016 study published in *Annals of Internal Medicine* did an intervention with 281 sedentary people who had excess weight or obesity, using behavioral-economics theory to assess exercise adherence. Lasting thirteen weeks, the goal was to get them to take seven thousand steps a day. The control group was given only daily feedback; the "gain" group got $1.40 for each day they *hit* the goal; and the "loss" group was *fined* $1.40 each day they *missed* the goal. There was also a lottery group that had the chance to win a small amount for hitting the goal.

The result? Fear of loss motivates best. The control group hit the target a third of the time; gain and lottery groups were 41 percent and 42 percent, respectively, and the loss group hit the step target 48 percent of the ninety-one days of the study. The latter also did better in the thirteen-week follow-up. These results lend support to the validity of prospect theory, which Kahneman expanded upon in *Thinking, Fast and Slow*, writing that we tend to weigh losses twice as much as gains.

Cass Sunstein, coauthor of the 2008 book *Nudge,* which Kahneman referred to as the "bible of behavioral economics," gave an apt example of how loss motivates more than gain in an editorial in *The New England Journal of Medicine* in 2015: "A 5-cent tax on the use of a grocery bag is likely to have a much greater effect than a 5-cent bonus for bringing one's own bag."

Risk vs. reward? The reality is, despite Resnicow's warnings, fear of loss can be a powerful motivator, especially for sudden change.

I was in despair prior to my life-changing epiphany. Why? Fear of loss.

Yes, I was in debt and engaged in unhealthy behaviors and was flunking out of school, but the larger issue was imagining how it would compound. I didn't despair over informing my parents near so much as I dreaded telling it to my straight-A pre-med girlfriend. I sensed it would spell doom for our relationship.

My love for her is a core value, and focusing on that made the change of my surface-level behaviors easy.

Chuck Gross worried over not being there for his child.

Lee Holland worried she'd coast through life without fulfilling her true purpose.

Josie Thomson *died*.

Avoiding negative consequences can be an initial motivator, but there is also positivity in change. For all of us, our lives became much better by this crystallization of discontent triggered by fear. Recall Rollo May: "One does not become fully human painlessly."

Perhaps you need to embrace that pain, acknowledge that fear, accept that guilt.

Guilt? Really? What about that self-compassion stuff? Yes, you can be compassionate regarding who you are, but that doesn't mean you've always done the right thing, both for yourself and for others. Acknowledging your bad decisions is one step in resolving not to repeat them. Yelling at your kids is an action. Loving them with all your heart is a core value. Let the core values rule the actions by realizing that behavior isn't the person you are; it's not a reflection of your true self.

In 2014, Harvard University researchers found that inducing feelings of guilt could create more moral decisions in the future.

Geez, James. You're being a real friggin' downer here.

To repeat: anxiety triggers analysis. It is just more information getting filed away for your brain to begin processing. Imagining this negativity isn't what triggers sudden insight. It's prep work. It's not about dwelling, but avoiding avoidance. A pile of research reveals that avoiding one's problems, be they regarding mental or physical health, employment or financial issues, or trauma (especially using drugs and alcohol as part of that avoidance), makes things worse, not better.

Negative emotions are evolutionarily adaptive. They have survival value by letting us know something is wrong; they're not something to be buried. You can't avoid such feelings, but you can seek to understand and learn from them. As wonderful as the life-changing epiphany sounds, it's not going to help solve your problems unless you first work on coming to terms with those problems. You don't have to go it alone. Friends, family, or therapy can all be beneficial allies in your struggle.

A holy-shit moment can be amazing, but it takes more than a snap of the fingers to make it appear. Remember, you can only coax the cat. Do the prep work, because when the prep work is done and we're distracted from our troubles and in a more positive mood state, then epiphany is most likely to strike with a massive "Hell, yeah!" Even if it never does, you'll still be better off for having done these exercises. And it may not be "never." The flash of insight might not happen this year but five years from now.

To paraphrase another Indiana Jones character (Belloq): Epiphany is not an exact science. It does not deal in time schedules.

Your task for this section is to consider risks and rewards. What are the potential negative outcomes of your current path? Are there health consequences? Could you be headed for financial ruin? Will your relationship last? Will your children dump you in some cockroach-infested nursing home? Will the police knock on your door? The behaviors you engage in today are paying off in some way, otherwise you wouldn't be doing them, but you need to do some long-term, consequence-oriented thinking.

Development of type 2 diabetes could mean losing a foot. Look at your feet. Which one do you want to keep? I'm guessing both.

Yeah, all that shit's a downer.

Do it anyway, and file it away. No need to dwell too much. It just needs to get processed for rumination.

Also consider the good side: the reward of positive change. Do that too. What are the beneficial outcomes that would result from taking action to avoid those losses?

Merge this with consideration of your real self; wait for lightning to strike.

Actualize This

I have to go to the bathroom.

That one is right at the base of American psychologist Abraham Maslow's hierarchy of needs, first published in 1943. It's a physiological demand that *must* be fulfilled. Excretion ranks on the same level as thirst, sleep, eating, breathing. . . . Above that in the hierarchy we have a need for safety (security, money, shelter, etc.), then love and belonging, then self-esteem-based needs. At the higher levels, the needs are more cognitive in nature. At the top is "self-actualization," fulfilling your personal potential.

Admittedly, modern psychology doesn't haven't much use for the hierarchy, and the term "self-actualization" has been used to sell pseudoscientific self-help books, retreats, and "universities" from gurus who will try to motivate you down to your last dollar. Like with "quantum," just because it's been misused doesn't mean the concept of fulfilling your potential lacks value. It still falls under "be the person you're meant to be."

You are not a blank slate. Almost thirty years after developing the hierarchy, Maslow wrote, "we already have capacities, talents, direction, missions, callings." The job, he explained, is to be more perfectly what you already are. It's worth noting that Maslow was keen on the phenomenon of the life-changing epiphany, referring to them as "peak experiences."

Despite how hard I dumped reality on you in the previous section, this doesn't have to be an endless cycle of embracing the suck of adulting. While *dwelling* on fantasy is unhelpful because of its demotivating qualities, you can still dream.

Gabriele Oettingen cautions in *Rethinking Positive Thinking* that we can become so attached to the comforts of positive thinking it loosens our grip on reality, compromising our ability to generate solutions to problems. But! "Positive fantasies may actually help you become *more* in tune with what is real, not less." The reality she mentions is digging in to what you really want.

I admit it. My wife and I watched that cheesy *Lucifer* show. Sue us.

The main character did this thing to get people to tell him their deepest wants. I'm not as good-looking or charming as actor Tom Ellis, and I lack his delightful British accent, but tell me, what do you truly desire?

Think on that for a moment while I drop a bit more science, then we'll get to your task for this section.

Oettingen asserts that "fantasizing is a powerful means of exploration." It allows you to engage in a virtual reality tour of a potential outcome without having to make a commitment. One example she uses in her book is a college student bound for medical school because it's what their parents did. But when the student creates a mental movie of all the micro details of what such a vocation looks like, and how this is in conflict with the student's personality, it reveals medicine as a poor career choice.

I've often been told I have a dream job, and I do love it, but it's still a job. Nothing is as glamorous inside as the outsider imagines. The majority of my job is sitting alone, at home, in sweatpants, writing silly sentences. It gets tiresome and lonely.

Self-actualization or no, *everything* is toil. But there are goals for which the pursuit—challenging as it may be—is an amazing experience, an amazing life.

Dream big, my friend, but sweat the small stuff of those dreams proactively so you choose well. Being a doctor isn't like it is depicted on *Grey's Anatomy*. I mean, I'm assuming it's not. I've interviewed a couple of stars from that show, but I've never seen it. Anyway, you know how System 1 constructs the story, and System 2 believes it? System 2 needs to do conscious work *first,* in most cases, for System 1 to come up with a good story to which the "slow" system of thinking can then say, "Yeah, we're down with that," because it already comprehends a lot of the details and is able to give quick confirmation.

Rage to Master

"Passion has no expiration date."

The previous sentence is the words of cognitive psychologist Scott Barry Kaufman in his book *Wired to Create.* I recommend Kaufman's book. It's rather how-to in nature; I consider it complementary to *The Holy Sh!t Moment.*

Kaufman speaks of falling in love with your dream via a crystallizing experience, because such crystallization does not have to focus solely upon discontent. My life was pretty good before I was driven to become a writer, but all those history papers and a master's thesis and strategic plans and business cases made me realize I had a skill I could transform into a career I was passionate about.

Like Maslow said, "We already have capacities, talents, direction. . . ."

Kaufman writes of the "rage to master," in which you have a skill that inspires you with "an intense and sustained drive for excellence." This can manifest in any way you please: parenting, gardening, fitness, cooking, accounting, poetry, music. . . . It is *your* life, and you can delve into those capacities and find your calling. If it's marketable, it can become a career. If not, it'll be a hobby you're passionate about. Or perhaps it's a way of living that brings joy to you and others.

In her book *The Happiness Project,* Gretchen Rubin writes, "Most decisions don't require extensive research," but Scott Kaufman countered with "Inspiration favors the prepared mind." He explained, "A focus on learning and growth increases the likelihood of being inspired, and in turn, inspiration leads to even higher levels of expertise." Inspiration and effort reinforce each other.

Capacities. Talents. Direction. Missions. Callings.

What are yours?

Socrates was pretty dark when he spoke of life not being worth living if you don't examine it. Not sure I buy into that. But a thorough examination can take your mind in the direction it needs—preparing it for inspiration—so epiphany doesn't just strike, the *right* one does.

Examine your life.

And it will never be the same, because when epiphany arrives, the real self and all its accompanying values of your true identity are unleashed from the false cage you constructed around it to get through each day.

The real self isn't just about a solitary purpose in life. There are many complementary drives you may come to possess. You can be multipurpose. You can be the Swiss Army knife of purpose-driven people.

Then you get to live the life you felt you were always meant to.

Determine Your Self

Women should do a breast self-exam. Men should examine their testicles. Unless you're me and married to a physician, then you can . . . Never mind.

How does one do a self-examination? Not of a body part, but a self-exam of the *self*? Self-determination theory (SDT) can help.

Self. Self. Self. Now it sounds weird.

Psychologists Richard Ryan and Edward Deci, both professors at the University of Rochester, codeveloped SDT, and they're big into the *eudaimonia* stuff mentioned earlier. In 2008, the two authored an article in the *Journal of Happiness Studies* contrasting hedonia with *eudaimonia*. The "hedonistic tradition" is a focus on the presence of positive effect and absence of negative effect, but *eudaimonia* is "living life in a full and deeply satisfying way."

The authors contend that just because someone is "happy," hedonistically speaking, doesn't mean they're psychologically well. *Eudaimonia*, conversely, is about actualizing your potential—the Maslow stuff: fulfill those virtuous potentials and live your life as inherently intended.

"Inherently intended" is loaded. Let us examine further.

"I believe there is something in there," Kennon Sheldon, professor of psychological sciences at the University of Missouri and an expert in SDT, told me. "There is personality. There is developmental potential. There are implicit interests; things that may have always been in there the person has not yet discovered. It is something to be awakened."

That's pretty deep. *Something to be awakened.* I can dig it. When I started going to class and paying attention, I gravitated to military history not because I was fascinated with who spilled whose blood on which battlefield, but because writing history papers—the composing of stories, even as academic analysis—felt so right to me. I'd been waiting to unleash that talent all my life, it seemed. I later completed a master's thesis examining American strategic containment of communism during the Cold War, and I aced that sucker.

Back to *eudaimonia.* It's related to autonomy, a fundamental psychological need central to SDT. (The two other aspects of the theory are relatedness and competence.) Simply put, SDT is about the intrinsic-extrinsic motivational spectrum.

Intrinsic motivation implies internal. You do something because it's fun; you derive pleasure or satisfaction from the activity itself. Intrinsic motivation is high in self-determination. As you slide down the spectrum, the degree to which the type of motivation is self-determined goes down.

The next four aspects of SDT are all forms of *extrinsic* motivation, having an external source. The first and most self-determined is "integrated regulation." This is behavior that confirms your sense of self (I am a writer/father/husband/exerciser—this is what I do). This is what motivated Chuck Gross toward his epiphany; he had the role of "dad" thrust upon him, creating a sudden shift in identity and values. Speaking of values, I place honesty over that of wealth, which is why I haven't packaged my neighbor's dogshit into gelatin capsules to sell over the internet as an all-natural miracle-weight-loss appetite suppressant.

"Identified regulation" follows, which is being motivated by goals *you* choose, such as losing weight, running a marathon, achieving status, higher learning, etc. Next is "introjected regulation," which comes from self-imposed pressure, such as refraining from drinking because you feel guilty over your intake. Finally, there is "external regulation," which is about obtaining rewards, such as money or praise, or avoiding punishment, such as loss of employment or being chastised.

Which one do you use? Answer: all of them.

My friend Steven M. Ledbetter is a behavior-change consultant and the CEO of Habitry. He refers to motivation as "painting a picture with several colors." Many assert that intrinsic motivation is "best," but Ledbetter considers that an oversimplification. "It's like saying breathing is better than your heart beating," he said. "People do things for *all* the reasons, intrinsic and extrinsic. There isn't a dividing line."

I obtain pleasure from the act of writing (intrinsic motivation). Writing is part of my identity (integrated regulation). I even dig the minor celebrity status (identified regulation). Considering my history, I don't wish to be viewed as lazy, so I work hard at it (introjected regulation). Finally, I liked getting both pay and praise for my work (extrinsic regulation). Like Steven said: *all* the reasons.

What's more, the primary motivator of any action can change from moment to moment. That being written, Ledbetter asserts that, over time, those who are more autonomous—more *self-determined* in their actions—have higher adherence rates.

Tying *eudaimonia* directly to SDT, in the same 2008 journal issue mentioned earlier, Ryan and Deci authored another piece showing how the two concepts are interconnected. Rather than looking at extrinsic goals focusing on wealth, fame, image, or power, the writers look at intrinsic ones, such as personal growth, relationships, community, and health. The authors assert that people who do so "behave in more prosocial ways, benefiting the collective as well as themselves." We are Borg. You will be assimilated. This caring for family and society beyond one's self strengthens your feelings of well-being.

It's feeling good vs. living well. Living well is about pursuing the *right* ends, engaging your best human capacities. This involves regular reflection and deliberation of your actions: the *examined* life.

And the holy-shit moment when epiphany strikes is often when we discover those right ends.

Professor Sheldon, using System 1 and System 2 descriptors, spoke of consciousness as "a bubble on the surface of the mind without much access to what's going on at deeper levels." But, he asserts, those deeper levels, the fast, System 1 unconscious thinking, holds a lot of information for us. "It may even be trying to break through."

Alas, we're often living a life not of our own making or choosing.

Sheldon explained that many of the goals we have are ones we feel we must, and we're pressured into pursuing them. Such demands can be societal or familial. Advertisements prompting you to consume also influence you. "You might even need therapy to furrow down and find out what these things are about," Sheldon said.

He wants you to cross the Rubicon.

We're getting into task stuff again. Please pay attention.

The goal is to pursue self-concordant goals, goals in line with who you are, your real self, and what you want to do with your life. Goals that are intrinsically satisfying and externally validating. The Rubicon metaphor relates to Julius Caesar's history-altering decision to cross that Italian river in 49 BC. Sheldon authored a paper (under review at the *Journal of Personality*) about self-concordant goals using this historical event as an analogy for when people cease deliberation and make their decisions, choosing to focus on specific goals to enact. At this point, "cognition shifts, from weighing information . . . to protecting and conserving the choice . . . and enacting plans to obtain that choice."

The promise is to take control of your future growth rather than "growing haphazardly . . . in reaction to accidents, stresses, or traumas." A source of guidance for making such a crossing is to examine your *potential* motivations for the various alternatives of where you go from here.

Take a moment and do that.

When faced with the various ideas of what You, Part 2 entails, ask tough questions about *why* you feel that way about each possibility. Is it because you think society expects it? Does family demand it? Or does it matter to *you*? Does it enrich who you are, allowing you to flourish, while also not being self-centered? In other words, does it have value for others as well? Especially those who matter to you most. Seek motivation that "feels right," Sheldon said.

When people examine potential motivation for a given path prior to making a choice, Sheldon's study revealed, it improves goal selection.

Do that. Look at the options and think hard about why you would choose them, then focus on the ones holding the most value for *you*.

How does one do that? There will be additional details regarding mindful meditation in chapter 9, but Sheldon asserts it's less about deliberation and more about *noticing*. Again, it's the distraction technique. You can belabor the question for a time, then give it a rest and let the answer float by. It may take some time.

Look for clues.

Professor Sheldon told me the story of Anna, a lawyer who was miserable. The name of an old friend, who Anna recalled had been a budding environmentalist, popped into her head. She looked up the friend and learned they were running an environmental firm and needed legal help. It completely changed her life for the better. Thinking of that friend was a message from the unconscious.

"If you have an open attitude toward your life, you can notice these hints," Sheldon said. And they can give you the power to be self-determined and truly inspired in your future endeavors.

Good to Great

I opened this book with a quote from Sir Winston, quoted him again earlier in this chapter, and am about to do it some more. Why? Because there was greatness to him. After the Bible and William Shakespeare, Churchill is the most frequent source of quotations. Because, damn, some of them are good. Like this one:

"To improve is to change, so to be perfect is to have changed often."

Winston was a soldier who saw battle on four continents, narrowly escaping death three times. He was an artist, sportsman, and statesman. He had more words published than Dickens and earned more royalties from writing than Hemingway or Faulkner. Unlike most other politicians, Winston wrote all his own speeches. He won the Nobel Prize in Literature in 1953 for his lifetime body of work.

Churchill was a Renaissance man, and a man of his time. That second part is a nice way of saying "bigoted as all hell." He may have done great things, but he did many terrible things as well. Descended from the Dukes of Marlborough, he was privileged up the ass. My interest in him is his way with words:

"If the present tries to sit in judgment of the past, it will lose the future."

In other words, crystallizing discontent and examining that over which guilt is felt is not about being paralyzed with feelings of wretchedness. It's a learning opportunity. You can look upon past mistakes and misdeeds with self-compassion, moving into the future as a better person for it. Recognize you have self-worth; endeavor to be better.

Not just better, great.

Good to Great, authored by business consultant and Stanford University lecturer Jim Collins, is a best-selling book about companies that make the leap toward amazing success, and what they have in common. It was required reading for us MBA types.

Interestingly, much of it can be applied to individual human behavior to make a similar leap.

Because perhaps life is peachy, but feel the words of twentieth-century author and radio personality Earl Nightingale: "Most people tiptoe their way through life, hoping they make it safely to death."

Nightingale was one of the few who survived the sinking of the USS *Arizona* during the attack on Pearl Harbor in 1941. As a child during the Great Depression, he lived in a tent city. He understood the human desire for security. It's on Maslow's hierarchy, just above pooping and breathing.

You may be living a good life. You may be safe. Do you seek more? Do you seek greatness? Read on.

Collins opens *Good to Great* with a quote from Beryl Markham, an adventurer and trainer of race horses who was the first woman to fly solo east-to-west across the Atlantic: "That's what makes death so hard—unsatisfied curiosity." And yet, Gallup's 2017 *State of the American Workplace* report determined only one-third of U.S. employees feel engaged at work. Screw that. Adventure is out there!

William James asserted we use only the smallest fraction of our potential. It's only under certain circumstances of constructive stress or deep feeling when we tap into emotional reserves to strive for greatness.

You need to think like a boss. Part of doing so involves avoiding what Ellen Langer calls "self-induced dependence."

Langer published a study in 1978 in the *Journal of Personality and*

Social Psychology involving mathematical problem-solving while getting participants to question their competence. The subjects began working on these problems on equal footing. Later, some were given the title "assistant," and others, "boss."

Once given the subordinate title, assistants solved the problems only half as well as previously. This is because, as the Heath brothers write in *Switch,* they adopt a "fixed mind-set." They "believe that their abilities are basically static."

The fixed mind-set is that you are who you are and can't change that. Conversely, the "growth mind-set" believes that no matter who you are, you *can* change.

To achieve greatness, it helps to resist conformity.

A 2006 study by researchers at Arizona State University about "going along vs. going alone" opens with a quote from Mark Twain: "Whenever you find yourself on the side of the majority, it is time to pause and reflect." The study asserts, "People are heavily influenced by the actions and beliefs of others." Doing so is socially adaptive, allowing us to reach accommodation on matters of importance. Going along is both self-protective and beneficial for "mate attraction."

I get the desire-for-sex part, but don't forget the "make it safely to death" stuff. To stand out and achieve greatness on your terms, using your capacities and talents, you may need to go against conformist programming and be willing to do what others are not. You may have a good life, but the first sentence in Collins's book is "Good is the enemy of great." It's easy to settle, it is safe and secure, which is why so many do.

I want to relay some of the highlights from *Good to Great* that apply not just to corporations but to your corporeal being.

"Facts are better than dreams." Collins borrows this quote from Winston Churchill to explain how you need to create a climate in your mind for which truth is heard. Do this by leading with questions rather than thinking you already have the answer, engaging in self-dialogue and debate rather than trying to coerce yourself, and conducting "autopsies" without blame when things go wrong. This reiterates a bunch of what I wrote earlier. And it helped make billions for corporations. So . . . it's good advice.

Another tip from Collins: "Strip away so much noise and clutter and just focus on the few things that would have the greatest impact." In other words, be a hedgehog, not a fox. Wait, what?

It's a parable about how the fox sees the complexity of the world yet is scattered in its thinking. It keeps attempting crafty ways to make a meal of the hedgehog, who always uses the same simple strategy to avoid being transformed into fox feces: curl into a ball and present the spikes. Works every time. Hedgehogs aren't stupid: "They took a complex world and simplified it." The examples Collins provides of others who simplified the world with great success are "Freud and the unconscious, Darwin and natural selection, Marx and class struggle, Einstein and relativity."

Taking this a step further, Collins examines the "Hedgehog Concept." It's a Venn diagram in which you find the intersection of three circles: What can you be best at? What are you passionate about? What drives your economic engine?

The last one may not apply, but in my case all three did when it came to a midlife career change. I saw no future in writing fiction because I wasn't that good, and there was little money to be made, but health-and-fitness writing presented numerous opportunities, and I sensed I could be better at it than most. As my career flourished, I realized the aspect I was most passionate about and had the talent to explore was the psychological side of the quest for excellence; the subject of motivation permeated my writing from the beginning.

Collins goes on to explain that we should not strive to be passionate about what we do but seek to do things we are passionate about. When we find our personal Hedgehog Concept, that which we feel destined to pursue, the author writes, there is a "ping of truth" to it. That ping is epiphany.

The book reaffirms much of what I've written: preserve your core values and chase "Big Hairy Audacious Goals." I'll wrap up my lauding of Collins's work with this quote: "The real question is not, 'Why greatness?' but 'What work makes you feel compelled to try to create greatness?'"

Before providing the anecdote for this chapter (and she's a delightful one), I want to give one more plug for rejecting that "safely to death" bullshit with another quote from Churchill: "It always looks so easy to solve problems by taking the path of least resistance. What looks like the easy road turns out to be the hardest and most cruel."

The cruelty being that you die, curiosity unsatisfied about the person you may have become.

Your next task is to ponder your Hedgehog Concept. We need to make some adaptations, however; you're a being, not a business.

What are you passionate about that compels you to create greatness? (No adaptation needed on this one.)

What can you be best at? This is on *your* terms. The corporate world is cutthroat, but you can choose goals that have rewards without need for comparison. Using your capacity and talent to flourish as an individual doesn't mean you must crush the competition. You may not need to engage in competition at all.

Finally, if it's career-oriented, what can you imagine that meets the two previous criteria *and* is marketable? Will it pay the bills?

Do that examination. Listen for the "ping of truth."

More than a Marathon Woman

On April 21, 2014, twenty miles into the Boston Marathon, I searched for my wife.

And there she was, right across from the Heartbreak Hill Running Company, just as we planned. I dashed over to the rail for several kisses.

When Kathrine Switzer, the first woman to officially run the Boston Marathon in 1967, tackled Heartbreak Hill the first time, she had no idea she was doing so; her mind was occupied with matters of greater import.

"My coach didn't believe a woman could run that distance," Switzer said. "When I told him Bobbi Gibb had jumped out of the bushes at the start to run the year before, he didn't believe it. I told him it was in *Sports Illustrated*!" Gibb was the first woman to run the course unofficially, in 1966. She had applied and received a rejection letter from the race director, who cited Amateur Athletic Union (AAU) rules that women were not allowed to run more than 1.5 miles competitively, because they supposedly couldn't handle the strain. Okay then.

Switzer was only twenty and thought she could just show up and run, but her coach, Arnie Briggs, insisted it be official. Switzer was a member of the AAU, and Briggs said she needed to follow the rules.

It was sheer luck she wasn't prevented from running.

Kathrine often used her initials, because she was tired of her first name being misspelled with an additional "e," and she was an aspiring writer who admired J. D. Salinger and thought "K.V." looked cool. She wasn't trying to break barriers, as Gibb had already run the race. She didn't realize it at the time, but Switzer is certain if she used "Kathrine" on the form, she'd have been rejected.

The other bit of luck was the freezing weather. She wasn't trying to hide, but the bulky tracksuit meant officials at the start line didn't realize a woman was about to run the race. The anonymity of her gender wouldn't last, however.

Race official Jock Semple saw Kathrine run by at the two-mile mark and became enraged. He attacked her, trying to rip the race bib that bore the number 261 from her chest, yelling, "Give me those numbers and get the hell out of my race!"

"I was blindsided by it," Kathrine told me. "I was terrified and yelled for help. I wanted to get away." Her boyfriend was running alongside and threw a shoulder into Semple, knocking him away. The photos of that moment would be seen around the world. To this day, they remain iconic.

But it nearly ended there. History was almost not made.

"My first instinct was to step off the course, because I was afraid and embarrassed," she said. Then she realized if she quit, people would say women are quitters, they can't do it. "I put my head down and decided I would finish on my hands and knees if that was what it took."

That was the first epiphany of the race for Switzer; the sudden realization that quitting wasn't an option. The larger epiphany that would forever change the world came eighteen miles later.

"Until that moment, I had been murdering Jock Semple in my mind," she said. "I kept wondering, *What is wrong with this guy?*" It was at mile twenty, the beginning of Heartbreak Hill, when her anger shifted.

She saw the faces of female spectators, some shone in approval and shouted encouragement, but many looked upon Switzer with scorn. "I was so disappointed more women weren't in the race." She wanted them to know how good running could feel. "I was mad at the women themselves," she said. "I thought it was their fault. Isn't that terrible?"

Kathrine didn't view herself as special; she became angry at her gender for believing those myths about female fragility. That was when the lightning bolt struck, a sudden insight that would define the next half century of her life and open running to women across the globe.

She suddenly realized how privilege had put her in that race. She was raised by parents who didn't discourage activity in girls but encouraged it; a rare upbringing in the fifties and sixties. That, and mentoring from Coach Briggs, made all the difference.

"Then I felt really stupid," Switzer said of the sudden understanding most women didn't have the opportunities she had. But the epiphany didn't stop there. Her mission in life awakened in a moment.

"Women had been discouraged all their lives, and I had been *encouraged*," Switzer said. "Running wouldn't even occur to them. It wasn't in their realm of consciousness." Her mission was to become the encouragement for them, to provide them the same opportunities she had. She didn't know what it was going to look like, or how she would accomplish such a thing to get women not just running, but running marathons, but she was suddenly determined.

"I *knew* I was going to find a way. There was no doubt in my mind."

Part of her path involved getting faster. Her first marathon was completed in four hours and twenty minutes; she ran as much as one hundred miles per week to improve. She won the New York Marathon in 1974 and got a personal best at Boston in 1975 with a lightning-fast time of two hours and fifty-one minutes.

Kathrine was instrumental in women being permitted to run Boston in 1972 and was at the starting line that year with the five other women who met the men's qualifying standard. That same year she helped organize the first women's road race in Central Park; seventy-eight women showed up.

Her greatest achievement was helping get the women's marathon into the 1984 Olympic Games in Los Angeles.

When Kathrine first ran Boston, the longest distance for women in the Olympics was only 800 meters. Men had been running the 26.2 miles in the Olympiad since it entered the modern era in 1896, and Switzer was determined to give women this opportunity as well.

Despite eight modern decades of male Olympic marathons, the barriers for women remained substantial. It was no longer about changing running in the United States, but worldwide, in countries where women's sporting events didn't even exist.

"They tried to convince me not to organize it. To me, it was as important as getting women the right to vote." The vote is about intellectual and social acceptance, Kathrine explained, and the marathon is physical acceptance.

Beyond the empowerment that running entails, it also provides access to education via athletic scholarships, another thing lacking for women in 1967. To this day, Kathrine Switzer helps organize women's running clubs around the world via her 261 Fearless organization, paying homage to the Boston Marathon bib number Jock Semple attempted to tear from her chest.

Speaking of Semple, they made peace, even became friends.

Kathrine ran Boston in 2017, on the fiftieth anniversary of her world-changing run, alongside thousands of other women she helped inspire and create opportunities for. After seventy laps around the sun, she crossed the finish line of the Boston Marathon once again.

Of the joy she felt, she said, "At that point, I felt like I could have run forever."

Life Spillage

Seen on Facebook; a haiku about getting out of bed:

No No No No No
No No No No No No No
No No No No No

It's early. The alarm goes off and shocks you into semiwakefulness. Who do you want to be?

Do you wish to be the person who rises to join the fray, excited about what the day will bring, or the one who says, "Aw, crap!" and hits the snooze button five times? My daughter, the straight-A student who kicks international ass at karate, repeatedly hits snooze. Her room is down the hall, and after the fourth time I find myself yelling, "For shit's sake, kid! Get the hell out of bed! Today is the one day I get to sleep in, and your stupid alarm clock is ruining it!"

Okay, bad example.

"Difficulties mastered are opportunities won."

Guess who? Yup. Churchill. Not done with him yet.

Say you have an epiphany, and it drives you to accomplish something awesome. The awesome doesn't stop with that one thing. There are cascade effects. There is spillover into other areas of life.

Nathan DeWall ran the Badwater 135 the week before I interviewed him. That's 135 miles. Through a place with the name Badwater. Running.

DeWall is our ass-kicking anecdote for chapter 9. For this chapter, he's another expert source, what with the whole psychology-professor-at-University-of-Kentucky-expert-in-self-regulation thing he has going on. As a teaser, it was a holy-shit moment that prompted him to go from a nonrunner to completing "Holy crap I can't believe I did that" distances.

We discussed the topic from both personal and professional perspectives. And at the simplest, hack-your-mind level, DeWall told me of a trick to exert greater self-control.

DeWall referenced a study published in 2011 in the *Journal of Research in Personality*. A method employed with participants was to get them to always use their nondominant hand for everyday tasks: carrying books, brushing teeth, cooking, and eating. "What they found is doing something like that gives you better self-control in other areas of life," he said.

It works well with aggression; you're less likely to lash out if you've been practicing using your nondominant hand. The self-control learned in one area spills over. Not only that, it seems to work best in those who need it most.

DeWall said becoming a dedicated ultradistance runner had numerous benefits both for family and work life. The discipline and time-management skills he developed were helpful, and his mood and focus improved as well.

Conquering obstacles to get good at one thing, and having that echo with other positive effects, is known as a "keystone habit."

Pulitzer Prize–winning investigative reporter for *The New York Times* Charles Duhigg writes of keystone habits in his book *The Power of Habit*. In it he tells the story of the Aluminum Company of America; how it was struggling in 1987, then the company's board of directors brought in Paul O'Neill as CEO to turn things around. His strategy: make it the safest company in America; zero injuries.

O'Neill announced his strategy at an investor's meeting, making no mention of improving profits or lowering costs. They thought he was crazy, but the new CEO's focus on achieving a specific area of excellence had tremendous spillover; the company thrived, including financially, as a result.

Success has a ripple effect. I've often extolled the virtues of physical activity not just for achieving fitness, but because of the proven benefits in myriad other aspects of life. I've written columns for the *Los Angeles Times* and *Chicago Tribune* investigating how being active improves cognitive capabilities, assists with alleviating depression, improves sleep, helps in cancer-treatment recovery, improves your odds of beating addiction, increases earning potential, decreases stress, enhances creativity, decreases disability, and alleviates pain.

In self-determination theory, development of excellence in one area can lead to "global motivation": you aren't lacking in drive to complete most of your day-to-day behaviors. Except for cleaning bathrooms. I don't know anyone who gets excited about that.

Chuck Gross despaired at his situation; but after his epiphany, not only did he lose half his body weight, he attained the ambition to get out of debt and go back to school to finish his degree, where he was a straight-A student. Formerly shy, he also gained confidence in his interpersonal dealings. Later, he became a competitive longsword fighter.

Josie Thomson found the strength to live a life of her own choosing, to question what she'd been taught, and to find her way in life exploring and creating her own belief systems. As a result, she's had a successful career and found true love and happiness. She left obedience to the ideals of others behind, gaining her independence.

We're not just talking about adopting new habits, but about life-changing epiphanies. And it's rarely about one thing when that happens.

"For most people, it wasn't about changing a particular behavior," William Miller said. Instead, it was about a shift in values. From his 2004 study published in the *Journal of Clinical Psychology*: "A common response, when we asked people what had changed, was 'everything.'"

Rebel or Revolutionary?

"The capacity to be disobedient is a marker of optimal health," Scott Kaufman told me.

But disobedient in the right way. A rebel just fights; a revolutionary initiates change. Kaufman suggests being disobedient in terms of not blindly playing by the rules and not always listening to what everyone else is telling you without thinking it through for yourself.

An epiphany that compels you to break rules *can* change you for the better, and the world along with it. Is altruism real? If everyone wins, does it matter?

Speaking of which, I didn't finish all the leftover Indian food. I saved half of it for my son.

I'm not a monster.

Act Now!

- Investigate who you truly are. Who is your real self? What are your core values? What is most important to you in life?
- Ask yourself what are the risks of your current path? Are there negative health consequences? Are you headed for financial ruin? Losing your mind in a soul-destroying vocation? Is your relationship on the rocks?
- Imagine the benefits of altering your path. Investigate some of the good that could come from inspired change.
- What are your capacities and talents? What do you think could be your true calling? Dig deep to better understand

what perhaps you were meant to do vs. what you're currently doing.

- Looking at your future alternatives, examine your *potential* motivation for each. Ask what you feel about the various possibilities and focus on ones that are about you flourishing as opposed to the objectives you feel thrust upon you from an outside source.
- Imagine your Hedgehog Concept: something you are passionate about that compels you to create greatness, something you can excel at, something that, if relevant, can pay the bills.
- Listen for the "ping of truth."

PART TWO

Epiphany and the
Emotional Self

WHAT'S GOING ON IN THERE?: THE BRAIN SCIENCE OF THE HOLY SHIT MOMENT

There is nothing better when something comes and hits you and you think "YES!"

—J. K. ROWLING

My daughter had a bearded dragon who was too stupid to live.

Evolution set this thing's brain to "zero." Considering how much loving care he required to prevent him from becoming fertilizer for our garden, I'm amazed such creatures ever made it out of prehistoric times alive.

His diet included live crickets, which had a tendency to escape and hide in every corner of the house then begin chirping up a storm. I had to send the kids out on seek-and-destroy missions to get some peace. Spiky—reptiles with spikes owned by little girls are always named Spiky—had a tendency to go into what the bearded dragon owner's guide referred to as "a state of semihibernation," in which they just stop giving a shit about living; they won't eat or drink and need to be coaxed back to health.

During one such episode, my wife and children were away, and I was left in charge of reptilian convalescence. I had to squirt baby food into his mouth, and like with a human baby, I'm not sure how much got in there. He also needed a bath, not to get clean, but to rehydrate.

Are you familiar with the expression "Is a frog's ass watertight?" It's akin to "Does a bear shit in the woods?" Well, a frog's backside may indeed keep water from entering, but such is not the case with a bearded dragon. The bath would allow him to soak up water via various avenues, so to speak.

I put him in the tub for a while, and he drank some, then began wigging out, so I took him out and dried him off.

It wasn't long before I noticed there was a problem.

Spiky couldn't walk.

Normally, he would lift his belly and tail off the ground and trot around, but he couldn't lift himself. He just flailed his legs and stayed in one spot, suffering some kind of reptile dysfunction. At this point, I recalled junior high school science class teaching us about one of the dumber dinosaurs—the stegosaurus—which was so stupid it needed a second brain in the back to control its hindquarters.

Well, that's just great, I thought. *I drowned his ass brain.*

Fortunately, it was temporary. Spiky lived a long life, despite his lack of cognitive capabilities.

Your brain is far more advanced than that of a bearded dragon. The human neural processing unit has immense capability for reflection, insight, and creative thought. And creativity is an important aspect in achieving a holy-shit moment. How do you imagine your way toward a life-changing epiphany? Let's peek under the hood. . . .

You can end up thinking of some interesting things when you're not trying to think about things. Stuff just pops in there. Just as I was preparing to write this chapter, a new article (new in November 2017) was published in *Frontiers in Psychology,* hypothesizing we don't have conscious thoughts. (I've met people like that.) At least, not directly. Rather than being top-down processing, it's bottom-up. The unconscious creates thoughts and emotions, and we consciously "become aware" of them. That's because the unconscious has access to everything, including the conscious mind.

The authors assert that consciousness is analogous to a rainbow: "It accompanies physical processes in the atmosphere but exerts no influence over them." Consciousness is an end-product, a way to broadcast what nonconscious executive systems came up with internally.

Far out.

To be clear, the authors do not dispense with free will, choice, or personal accountability. It's more about how the human brain is so complex that there is a lot of stuff going on behind the scenes that rules behavior we aren't even aware of. Daniel Kahneman addressed this in *Thinking, Fast and Slow*. We think we know what's going on in our minds: one conscious thought leading to another in an orderly manner. Except most stuff arrives in our thoughts without us knowing how it got there. We allow ourselves to be guided by impressions and feelings without even realizing we're doing it.

A 2010 review article in *Trends in Cognitive Sciences* asserts that the primate brain is an interconnected, large-scale network that evolved this way as a survival mechanism to "accommodate a wide variety of environmental contingencies." At any moment, dangerous things can happen, and if you don't respond the correct way, you get dead and Charles Darwin laughs at you. Perceptions and learned concepts and understanding of the environment all must fire rapidly to create an immediate solution. Otherwise, Elton John is going to sing that circle-of-life song again.

Researchers were examining the phenomenon of automatic behavior even prior to the twentieth century. Famed novelist and poet Gertrude Stein even got in on it (she was a student of William James's in her younger years). Together with her coauthor Leon Solomons, the pair published a study in *Psychological Review* in 1896, revealing how body movements often take place without conscious control, including the acts of reading and writing. More than a century ago, scientists were examining how memory and habit create both action and thinking beyond conscious control.

That being said, Kounios and Beeman write in *The Eureka Factor* that there is no scientific consensus that "unconscious thought" exists. It might be a particular type of complex problem-solving that takes place "outside of awareness." The authors contend there isn't an *Austin Powers* Mini-Me inside your brain doing the work for you while you play golf. It's still *you* who is thinking, automatically, without realizing you're thinking.

I think my brain hurts now.

Sometimes we methodically arrive at an answer to a challenging problem via steady, linear analysis. Other times, stuff pops in, seemingly out of nowhere.

And technology allows us to examine what it looks like in the brain when that happens.

Insight Out

"An insight doesn't always occur as a scientific breakthrough," Professor Mark Beeman told me. "Sometimes it's about how you are going to organize your closet."

Next, we talked about life insurance.

Back in 2009, Mutual of Omaha launched a campaign referring to the company as "Proud sponsor of life's aha moments." I guess it had something to do with meditation and inspiration: "Om!" and "Aha!" creating "Omaha," because they wanted to take people's minds off the fact Nebraska is a place that exists.

For years, they collected video stories of people telling about their aha moments as part of an advertising campaign. A 2015 video compilation showed various individuals talking about their sudden insights: "You can set fear aside," and "The change starts in your head," and "There's a moment when you just know," and "You never know when that one moment is going to change your life and affect so many other people."

They may have sponsored life's aha moments, but they had no interest in putting money toward laboratory study of the phenomenon. Mutual of Omaha referenced Kounios and Beeman's work in the campaign, but when the pair asked if the insurance company would be interested in funding research, it was Mutual of Tumbleweeds.

The videos are still cute and show the myriad forms of how life can change in a moment.

"Sometimes we just fumble our way along and never do solve the problem of 'What should I do with my life?'" Beeman said. He explained life is just another set of information people are trying to organize and understand, and sometimes it feels like it's all set out before them, and they follow from one thing to another, failing to ask themselves the big questions. But for those who do, it's a complicated process of attempting to organize your life around certain principles, especially when you're not sure what those principles are.

"But the information is there." Sometimes you don't know it's a problem, but you feel something is wrong, or there is a puzzle to be understood. We get bits of feedback here and there that suggest we are unhappy with the status quo, we just haven't put it into a global context yet.

"A lot of people get to a point where it tips over," Beeman said. "Insight seems really important to motivational persistence." The knowing of *rightness* is motivating all by itself.

It's the "ping of truth" thing.

How does your brain find that truth? Let's start with a bit of anatomy.

Introducing: Your Brain

Have I made you laugh? I mean, you're still reading, so hopefully not all my jokes fell flat.

If you chuckled, it was the left side of your brain comprehending the words I wrote, and the right side that got the joke. Even if you groaned and rolled your eyes—right side. The starboard hemisphere of USS *Noggin* has access to broader neural networks allowing it to be more flexible in the understanding of the information that's coming in. It's less bound to literal thinking; it's more responsible for the creation of epiphany.

More responsible, not solely. The left uses the slower, System 2 manner of thinking, and the right uses the faster, System 1. More or less. The two sides aren't like one of those marriage-gone-bad couples who got divorced and now they never talk. The corpus callosum facilitates communication between the two hemispheres, and in a much more cooperative way than divorce lawyers do. What's more, the brain has plasticity, especially while young, to remodel itself if necessary.

An extreme example of such plasticity is children with Rasmussen's encephalitis, a rare inflammatory disease that causes severe and debilitating seizures. In some cases, treatment involves hemispherectomy.

If that word makes you cringe, it should. It involves removing one side of the brain. The *entire* side.

What's fascinating is the research showing that children who have undergone this procedure can regain much of their language ability after having the left hemisphere removed (or disconnected), because the right hemisphere adapts in its absence.

Digging deeper into the gray matter, you have the frontal lobe, which is, well, at the front. It's involved in problem-solving: setting goals, planning, decision-making, etc. It helps narrow focus, so you don't get paralysis via analysis. But that also creates problems when it comes to insight: it limits possibilities.

In 2005, researchers at the International School for Advanced Studies in Italy looked at people with drain bamage. I mean brain damage.

I am going to hell.

Anyway, the researchers presented thirty-five patients with frontal lobe damage with insight problems and compared them against a control group of twenty-three participants who had no such damage. The results? Those with lesions on the frontal lobe solved the most difficult insight problems at almost twice the rate of the healthy participants (82 percent success rate vs. 43 percent). This is because the frontal lobes "bias" your response space. As Kounios and Beeman assert, while the frontal lobe is engaged in important cognitive functions, it is also a "jailer that keeps us trapped in the box."

Your next task is to locate a suitably sharp implement, ensure it is well sterilized, and stab—On second thought, there is a less invasive way to expand your mind that allows you to retain those important executive functions the frontal lobe is responsible for.

Keep reading. Not just this book. But lots of things. Keep thinking too. Expand your expertise. Continuously. Grow your mind through practice. Kounios and Beeman explain how your past informs your beliefs, assumptions, and expectations while also limiting the flexibility of your thinking. "We continuously build mental models of the world around us—our boxes—to help predict what will happen next." They refer to the brain as an "anticipation machine," and this can create tunnel vision.

But a wealth of experience grows the box. It creates a greater breadth of possibility and opportunity. Growing your knowledge base is part of the coaxing of the cat. As mentioned with chaos theory, you need to do different things to create different outcomes. Except this isn't the butterfly effect, it's expanding understanding so the box is bigger, the tunnel wider, the opportunities for epiphanies more expansive in nature, because your brain sees more, understands more, and can conceive of greater possibilities.

Finally—well, not *finally,* because there is a metric shit-ton of brain stuff we won't examine—there is the anterior cingulate. It does . . . a lot of stuff.

Your brain is pretty awesome, but it's still limited, both in speed and power. That's why I can't remember what it was I got up and walked into the other room to do once I arrived there. The anterior cingulate is a prioritization machine, because your brain can't make *all* the calculations based on *all* the data the way a supercomputer does. It engages in "triage" based on the "emotional value" of information.

Which ties back to the rider and elephant. Told you it was important to feel this.

It's because of the anterior cingulate that mood affects insight, as we'll learn more about later in this chapter. Prior to getting into that, let's see how the brain deals with rodents.

The RAT and Your Brain

Hopefully that subtitle doesn't trigger cold sweats because you recalled some horror movie about brain-eating zombie rats. There are no actual rodents. It's an acronym for Remote Associates Test; we touched on it earlier with the research regarding how exercising outdoors enhances creativity. Using RAT is how the researchers tested the boost in creative ability.

Pine. Sauce. Crab.

What one word fits all three? What can you remotely associate?

There are two ways to approach it: analytically, or via the *poof* method.

Got it yet? If yes, how? Did you methodically test words, eventually finding one that fit with pine, sauce, and crab? Or did the answer pop in out of nowhere? Or were you testing words, then you suddenly had the answer, and you knew it was right without having to test it? Those latter two qualify as insight.

Apple. If you haven't gotten it yet, the answer is apple.

If you were testing words, I bet one of the first ones you thought of was "tree," yes? It works for two of them, but even though maple syrup is awesome stuff, no one refers to it as "tree sauce."

For years prior to writing *The Eureka Factor,* Kounios and Beeman conducted numerous studies, using EEG and fMRI technology, to see what goes on inside the brain when sudden insight arrives.

EEG refers to electroencephalography. That's John Kounios's domain. It provides temporal information. Don't think "temporal lobes," think *Star Trek.* "Captain, I'm detecting a temporal displacement; we seem to have traveled back in time to the 2016 U.S. presidential elec—" *"REVERSE THRUSTERS!"*

So, yeah. "Temporal" refers to time. It provides precise information about *when* a specific brain activity takes place. This is coupled with fMRI, functional magnetic resonance imaging (Beeman's area of expertise), for the spatial data—*where* the brain is activated.

You could say this combination of technologies reveals the space-time continuum of the brain.

Back to more earthbound studies. Subjects were given the RAT—presented with three words, not furry little vermin—and told to press a button immediately upon thinking of the word that fit all three. They were not to take time to verify the solution. Then they were asked to verbalize the solution and press another button to indicate if the solution was achieved via sudden insight or via methodical testing of various words until finding one that fit.

When the solution arrived via sudden insight, the EEG showed a rapid surge of gamma waves. "We were amazed at the abruptness of this burst of activity," the authors write. It was, however, just what they expected from a sudden insight. At the same time, fMRI showed increased blood flow in part of the *right* temporal lobe called the anterior superior temporal gyrus. This part of the brain is involved in making connections between distantly related ideas, such as getting a joke or comprehending a metaphor. That part of the brain didn't light up when the solution was arrived at methodically.

I italicized the word "right" in the previous paragraph. Remember, insight is right-brain stuff. Except not totally.

Kounios and Beeman replicated the fMRI study using "more powerful procedures" and learned that the right temporal lobe isn't the only thing activated with sudden insight. Rather, "A whole network of brain areas is involved." The right temporal lobe activity was still most prominent, but their work reinforces earlier statements regarding how all types of thinking involve multiple aspects of neural processing across the brain.

Who cares? I want to have an epiphany so I can lose weight or quit drinking or go back to school or paint a masterpiece.

We're getting to something actionable here. Hang on.

Immediately prior to achieving sudden insight, there is a phenomenon called a "brain blink."

At the moment of insight, the EEG showed a massive burst of gamma waves. But for about one second beforehand, the brain emitted alpha waves. Alpha is slow; the neurons aren't processing information. If you imagine an automobile engine, the authors contend, "The car is working, but it isn't going anywhere. Alpha is a neuron's park."

The brain idles, ever so briefly, preparing for insight to strike.

Say I ask you a challenging question that requires a moment of thought. What will you do when I ask it? Will you look away from the distraction of the book for an instant? Perhaps close your eyes?

The reason you do this is because a large part of the brain is dedicated toward visual cognition. Vision can dominate our neural processes, making it more challenging to determine the answer to a difficult problem.

And the burst of alpha waves cuts off visual inputs for a moment, so you can better focus and achieve sudden insight. In a 2009 study published in *Current Directions in Psychological Science,* Kounios and Beeman discovered that when the brain is about to come to a solution via insight, brain activity directs attention *inward.* We're not looking to the outside world to find the solution; we are engaged in "retrieval." We already have it stored in the biological equivalent of RAM. The brain is using the anterior cingulate, which is involved in detecting weakly activated, subconscious solutions, to *neuro-google* the answer.

How is this actionable? It reinforces the diversionary aspect of racking one's brain until stuck, then doing something distracting to take your mind off it. Give your brain some peace so it can process the information.

This next part is cool.

"It turns out," Professor Beeman told me of the RAT studies, if subjects "came up with the answer by insight instead of analytically, their accuracy rate is much higher." Statistically and reliably over many studies, this was the case.

That doesn't mean it's an error-free system. Professor Daniel Kahneman was coauthor on a 2010 study published in *Trends in Cognitive Science* which asserted, "System 1 can generate complex representations, but it does not have the capability for rule-governed computations." System 2 is still required for validation, but it appears to have been involved in the computations all along, just unknown to the individual, because the sensation of rightness is immediate.

MAKE IT HAPPEN!

Pull out your phone and find some space in your calendar for ten minutes a day for the next few days to get used to trying this out. Put it in the actual calendar when you know you can take this ten minutes uninterrupted. And during those ten minutes, find a distraction-free environment. No phones or screens or books or music. Sit in a comfortable chair and let your mind wander about anything at all. Focus on nothing but your breathing for a time, then allow imagination to take you where it may. Think of an old movie or a new one. A book you read, the dreams of youth, a story someone told you. Jump from idea to idea. Reclaim the lost art of daydreaming with the knowledge that it's important to this process and the opposite of a waste of time. Do it guilt free as an endeavor in practicing self-care and achieving your utmost potential.

That's it. It's not meditation, but free association; fantasizing without structure or effort of will. You're not thinking about what to think about; let things flow in and out, naturally.

Get into a habit of doing this, and insight may arrive.

Instinct and Insight

Wolfgang Köhler was a twentieth-century German psychologist who contributed to the development of Gestalt psychology. He referred to instinct as a dynamic pattern, something arrived at after the failure of trial and error. When insight leads to a solution after such a failure, that solution is then applied to similar problems in the future, making insight learning an active process rather than a passive one.

It's not just a human behavior: Kohler observed it in chimps questing for a food reward. They would be provided food that was out of reach, attempt to reach it, and fail. Then the chimps would look around their environment, finding crates and sticks that would help them reach the food. Sudden insight gave them the ability to use these tools and commence shoving food in face holes.

Later, when presented with difficult-to-reach food, trial and error was skipped. They jumped straight to the insight-gained solution. This means they learned by perceiving the problem rather than focusing on the reward.

Mark Beeman echoed this for humans.

"We are starting to look at rewards for predicting insight. Turns out, it doesn't usually work." People lose focus when there is a reward. If it's presented subliminally, with a hint of a big reward, then they do better. This phenomenon is connected to the neurotransmitter dopamine, which we'll learn more about later in this chapter.

In 2007, Leonid Perlovsky, a visiting scholar at Harvard and a principal research physicist for the United States Air Force, prepared a report for the Air Force Research Laboratory, which explores how the knowledge instinct has driven the evolution of consciousness. Perlovsky asserts, "The two main aspects of the knowledge instinct are differentiation and synthesis." Differentiation is proceeding from less knowledge to more, and synthesis is understanding the meaning of that knowledge. *Emotional investment* is an aspect of synthesis: how we feel about information affects the meaning we take from it. And greater synthesis results in faster differentiation, "taking things from vague and unconscious states to more crisp and conscious states."

This is reminiscent of Immanuel Kant and his 1781 *Critique of Pure Reason*, in which he stated, "Thoughts without content are empty; intuitions without concepts are blind. . . . [O]nly from their unification can cognition arise."

After being successful, the chimps again get presented with hard-to-reach food, and they instantly know how to solve the problem. Even if the tools change, they can look around and see different boxes and sticks and think, *We can work with that.* There is an instantaneous *feeling* of rightness.

The research using remote associates tests confirms it: When we get the right answer to a problem via sudden insight, we don't have to double-check. We just know.

We just know because we've been there before. We may not recall solving these kinds of problems previously, but we have, and that's a big part of the reason *why* we know. Kahneman refers to the brain as "an associative machine." We don't run through a sequence of separate conscious ideas, one after the other. Rather, one idea activates others, which activates others, and so on. Only a few of them consciously register. Most of the work is silent, unconscious.

Your brain already has a ton of information to work with to reach epiphany. It's possible for you to have one today, after you set this book aside. Kathrine Switzer had hers at age twenty, while running Heartbreak Hill. As she said, she didn't know what the details would look like, but epiphany gave her a mission that April day in 1967, and it drove her, relentlessly, for the next half century.

Whether epiphany arrives soon or not, keep cramming ideas in there to increase the odds of the initial insight or the later, clarifying epiphanies to come. Grow the box of your thoughts. Widen the tunnel of your vision. Synthesize it all by examining how you feel about it.

That was another task, FYI.

A Dual Process

I am driving this point home one final time regarding how System 1 constructs the story and System 2 believes it. Why? Because it's not just System 2 that needs to do the believing, Indy.

You do, too.

Believe the cat can be coaxed by preparing System 2 with information, then creating the situations in which System 1 can do its thing.

The initial concept of dual-process theory dates to William James in 1890, who wrote of associative vs. true reasoning. In 2008, researcher Jonathan Evans, an emeritus professor of cognitive psychology at the University of Plymouth in England, wrote a review of the study into the dual-process model of cognition. "Almost all authors agree on a distinction between processes that are unconscious, rapid, automatic, and high capacity, and those that are conscious, slow, and deliberative."

Evans, using the terms popularized by Daniel Kahneman, looked at the labels attached to the two systems across the decades. System 1 is "Automatic/Experiential/Implicit/Associative/Intuitive/Reflexive," whereas System 2 is "Controlled/Rational/Explicit/Rule-based/Analytic/Reflective."

The author concluded the "generic dual-system theory is currently oversimplified." It's like the right brain, left brain stuff. There is crossover; it's not a sharp dividing line.

But does that matter to you? You're not looking to have research on this subject published in a peer-reviewed journal, are you? Simplification mixed with a bit of swearing is what I do.

So, really simply, once again, cram your brain with shit.

Good shit, though. Think about what you're going to do with the rest of your life. This life is the only one you have, and I don't recommend cruising the rest of your days on autopilot. What would things look like if you didn't tiptoe, but made some leaps, and one day, hopefully a long time from now, you made it *unsafely* to death? Rather than strolling, what if it was a thrill ride?

That's another task: think on the possibility.

The Post-Epiphany System

Eureka happened in a bathtub.

The "eureka," the one after which the word supposedly came to be popularized. I write "supposedly" because we are talking over a couple millennia ago, with the tale of Greek mathematician Archimedes.

Long story short, some king wanted to know if his crown was pure gold and asked Archimedes to figure it out. Density of gold is known, so he needed to determine the *volume* of the crown, without damaging it, to solve the problem.

One day, he stepped into the tub and saw how the water was displaced, realized he could use the same methods to determine the volume of the crown, and jumped out of the tub yelling, "*Eureka!*" which is ancient Greek for "I have found it!" According to the story, he even ran down the street, naked and dripping wet, yelling this. I like imagining that part as true, which is why the word persists to this day. A naked mathematician sprinting down the road yelling shit is going to leave an impression.

What happened next? I suspect he devised a method of immersing the crown to measure the displacement, then used that information, combined with the weight, to determine the crown's density, and told the king if he got ripped off or not.

All that post–jumping-out-of-the-tub stuff is System 2.

The moment of realization—the eureka—was System 1 generating the idea, while also getting that quickie confirmation from System 2, so Archimedes *knew* he had the solution, but the enactment of that solution relied on more analytical processes.

Scott Kaufman writes of this in *Wired to Create.* The spontaneous processes play the larger role in the "*generative* phase" of creativity—coming up with the idea in the first place—whereas more rational processes are at work during the "*exploratory* phase"—pondering enactment of the creative ideas you came up with.

In the Mood for Epiphany

If you started singing the above heading to the tune of Robert Plant's 1983 hit "In the Mood (for a Melody)," then I suspect you and I could be friends.

"When you let go," Professor Beeman told me, "you can see the big picture more clearly." A positive mood results in relaxation, which permits epiphany to strike. But perhaps "positive" isn't always the correct term. Sometimes it's about letting go.

Beeman and I spoke of the case of Wag Dodge. In 1949, he led a team of fifteen firefighters parachuting into Mann Gulch in Montana to battle a brushfire. The wind suddenly changed, and the fire raced toward the men. They attempted to climb up the side of the hill to outrun the fire, but Dodge knew it was hopeless. He was resigned. They were going to die.

Dodge ceased his futile flight; the others continued fleeing in terror. Wag was preparing to meet his maker when a sudden insight saved his life.

He took out a match and lit the grass in front of him. The wind blew the fire he created up the hill and away from the blaze chasing toward him, leaving a charred patch of ground. He crawled onto the newly created bare spot and waited as the fire burned around him.

He survived. Twelve of the other firefighters did not (two other survivors found safety from the flames via a rocky crevice at the top of the gulch). Had he continued his panicked flight, he never would have thought fire could be used to fight fire. Surviving required a relaxed state of accepting one's fate.

Recall how I talked about the anterior cingulate and its role in neuro-googling for subconscious, less obvious solutions to problems? It turns out that this part of the brain is activated by a positive mood and shut down by anxiety. Kounios and Beeman were able to test this by having participants watch different films. Comedies increase insight; anxiety-inducing films reduce it.

You can bet that bit of information will influence one of the tasks for this chapter.

Kahneman echoes Kounios and Beeman's research. When you're in a good mood, you trust your intuitions, but if you feel strained, "you are more likely to be vigilant and suspicious." You're more cautious because of the analytical mind-set, but less intuitive and creative.

Once again, this reveals the importance of the dual process. Analysis can be an important part of priming for epiphany.

Chuck Gross had been dwelling on his obesity for months. The pregnancy announcement was a great joy for him and triggered sudden epiphany.

Lee Holland was unfulfilled but riding high from having worked hard that day to help a man and his son in desperate need.

I was in a state of despair, yet not in that moment. I was chuckling over an amusing section of the school paper.

Except it may not be quite so simple as good vs. bad mood. In 2013, researchers from the University of New South Wales found it may be more about "motivational intensity" regarding broadening and narrowing one's cognitive scope. It's more like a state of relaxation. When you're scared shit-less because Jason Krueger is about to hand-machete the entirety of Crystal Elm Lake Street, it will narrow your focus. Alternatively, a good laugh over the antics of a hyperintelligent baby on *Family Guy* can chill you out. It's a worthwhile distinction to make. Earlier, I relayed research about "sudden gains" in alleviation from depression. You can't tell people with clinical depression to just get in a good mood to allow epiphany to strike, but it can be feasible for them to achieve a more relaxed, distracted state.

It's after epiphany strikes when motivational intensity explodes. It's the excitement of rightness, often mixed with the dramatic relief mentioned in chapter 1. That's what drives.

Rider and elephant, rationality and emotion, working together. Previously, we examined the identity-value model of self-control. In 2016, researchers from the University of Oregon analyzed several studies revealing that when people think about their identity and beliefs and values, brain imaging shows the ventromedial prefrontal cortex is activated.

This area of the brain is directly involved in the regulation of emotion.

Add to this research into people with lesions on the amygdala—a part of the brain necessary for processing emotion—who as a result had difficulty making decisions, and it further drives home the point.

It's not about hearing the "ping of truth." It's about *feeling* it.

Driven by Distraction

"Lose your mind and come to your senses," said Dr. Fritz Perls, a twentieth-century psychiatrist. He cautioned against turning into a total hippie burnout, however.

How to lose your mind effectively? "Shower thoughts" are a popular distraction technique referenced by Kounios and Beeman.

The pair write of how the water creates a white-noise effect. You can't focus on it, and it blocks out other sounds. The warmth of the water makes you comfortable. Sometimes your eyes are closed, cutting off those distracting visual inputs. The routine is automatic via years of practice. You are cut off from the environment; your brain can drift.

Mychelle Vega's life changed in the shower. Not just changed but was *saved*.

"I was replaying everything that had brought me to that exact moment," Mychelle said. "I realized I needed to break free of the soul-crushing, mind-numbing state of depression and despair I was in."

It was February 2013, and Mychelle was thirty-five years old. The comforting warmth of the water washed over her, making her pensive. She considered the trials of the previous three years. She grew up in Colorado, a place she loved, but had been laid off, had run out of money, and was dating a man who "was sucking the life out of me and leaving me as a shell." She felt she had no choice but to move to Atlanta to live with her grandparents. She didn't like the city and felt as though the family environment was "toxic." She often hid in her bedroom, living a life cut off from everyone, but she felt like she had no options.

She considered on a daily basis ways to end her life. Her mother had guns, her grandparents had pills. "It was a struggle to get out of bed and breathe.

"In the shower I had an epiphany that I had to get out. It hit me like a ton of bricks. I had to get back to Colorado, no matter what it took." It was that or die. "It was locked in. I couldn't go another day without moving toward this light at the end of the tunnel."

She spent the next ten days scrounging what little cash she had for gas money, mapping her route, arranging places to sleep along the way. "If I didn't have to spend money on something, I didn't." She ended up in Littleton, just south of Denver. She would park outside Starbucks and use their wifi to look for jobs. She stayed with friends and slept in her car until she got a temp job that allowed her to slowly improve her life.

Now Mychelle is happily married, working as an accountant, and getting a degree in business management at Colorado State University, all because of that snap decision in the shower, where the peace and calm let her see the way forward.

Once again, it's about the anterior cingulate. It's searching for those subtle, alternate possibilities buried deep in the unconscious. It needs peace and calm to find them.

"Anxiety is a good focused state," Beeman said. "But the problem is sometimes we focus on the wrong things, things that get in the way." After the anxious state, however, when we let go, "you can see the picture much more clearly." And being tired can help. A 2011 study of 428 students published in *Thinking & Reasoning* determined that one's ability to solve problems via insight peaks during "non-optimal times of the day." The study revealed we're about 25 percent more effective at using insight for problem-solving when fatigued. Of course, analytical ability takes a hit during this time, which is kind of the point. When we're tired, we're less inhibited; the analytical mind lets go, and tunnel vision is no longer an issue. Our minds are too exhausted from the day's mental labors and can flow into unforeseen areas because we lack the energy to restrict it.

Time for another task.

Work on analysis until the problem "sticks in your craw—and your brain." Then take a shower. Go for a walk outside. (No phone!) Watch a funny movie. Relax in a way that leaves your brain unoccupied. Beeman also suggests sleep.

Speaking of sleep, he told me the story of Otto Loewi.

Loewi was a German pharmacologist who, almost a century ago, had a dream. A literal one while he was asleep, not like the ones I had as a teen about the Dallas Cowboy cheerleaders and a desert island. Loewi awoke in the middle of the night, inspired about his research. He made some notes so he wouldn't forget, and went back to sleep.

And, dammit, the next day he couldn't read those notes. They looked like scribbles. The next night, the dream returned. Rather than chance writing it, he got up and went down to his lab to begin an experiment on how chemical substances affect neurotransmitters.

"That eventually led to him winning the Nobel Prize," Beeman said, finishing the tale.

He advises not just jumping out of bed when that alarm goes off. Rather, when you awaken, spend some time just lying there with your thoughts. See what enters your mind.

Work on your distraction techniques. Let the anterior cingulate be a search engine of the unconscious.

And lightning may strike.

Insight into the Truest Self

"We didn't believe there was any room for alternative lifestyles."

Josie Charlotte Ramsay lives outside Fargo, North Dakota. She was raised in a staunch Republican, Catholic family. "The church was a big part of my upbringing," she said. Another part of her upbringing was being raised as a boy.

"I was taught, especially by our faith, that homosexuality was wrong. My father made it clear boys were boys." But she didn't feel like a boy. She would walk around in her mother's shoes and have a feeling of rightness, only to be yelled at: "Boys don't do that stuff!"

She cross-dressed in secret through childhood. Josie had mental breakdowns due to being forced to deny who she was. She confessed to her priest, who said secretly wearing women's clothes was morally neutral but that she had to take care it went no further. She prayed to God every night to make her a girl. "I'd cry myself to sleep, but I'd wake up and still be a boy." Gradually, she lost her faith.

It was a continual cycle of wanting to express herself yet having it suppressed by her parents, her classmates, and the church. "I was told I would go to hell. It was devastating for my psyche."

She engaged in a behavior the trans community refers to as "purging."

"I would say, 'What the hell is wrong with me? I just need to be a man.'"
And all the clothes and makeup would be thrown away. "There was broiling self-hatred. I knew I was different and I didn't want to be." She wanted to be like her dad, a husband and a father, because "that's what you were supposed to do."

Because of the denial, the self-hatred, and the sheltered life, Josie didn't know who she was. She thought perhaps she was a cross-dresser. Other times, she imagined she was gay. It never occurred to her she was a woman.

She didn't have the term "transgender" in her mind. Her life was a mess, she said. She dropped out of school. Then she had the first of what she referred to as an "Oh, shit" moment.

"My brother and I were the only children. We loved each other so much." Her brother, Timothy, suffered kidney failure in January 2011, caused by a misdiagnosed fungal infection. She watched him die in the hospital, then sat with his body for three hours waiting for the coroner to arrive, who was late due to a snowstorm.

"Sitting there with him, it made me suddenly realize my self-image was artificially constructed," Josie said. She did not yet know who she was but realized who she *wasn't*. In her words, a layer of the onion peeled back.

"My life was on the wrong track." Living with her parents. Minimum-wage job. Dropped out of school three times. No direction at all. The sudden loss of her brother, and being there next to his lifeless body, opened her mind to the truth of the situation. Josie told me her brother had a fire to him, and in his memory, she made a reemergence. She would get out of this rut. It began by going out and making new friends. In doing so, she was drawn to women.

Because of her caring heart, it was suggested she try nursing school. In the female-dominated field, she flourished.

"One night, in the fall of 2013, they took me to a male strip show." She realized she was attracted to men, but not *as* a man. Whenever she tried to be romantic with a man, it didn't feel right. She didn't enjoy stubble on stubble. Another layer peeled back.

"I certainly wasn't there yet. I was still deep in denial, still living as a man." After graduating as a licensed practical nurse, she moved to Duluth,

Minnesota, a port city of eighty-five thousand people. Sharing an apartment with a very feminine woman, she said she never felt safer or more fostered. "I started occasionally dressing in female clothing again."

But denial persisted. Her upbringing would not permit her to think differently.

Early in 2015 she had a second, larger epiphany. She was at a bar in Duluth with her friend Chelsea. Called the Red Herring, it was, as Josie described, "an artsy bar, kind of new-wave." A DJ played electronic dance music.

Josie was dressed as a woman. "I felt more female than I ever had in my life."

That night, Chelsea made Josie face down her lifetime of denial. They sat together on a couch, and her friend said, "It doesn't matter if something is practical or not. *Life* isn't practical. You have to go forward as you really are." Chelsea gestured at Josie, indicating her clothing, hair, and makeup. "And *this* is who you are."

In an instant, after so many years of suppression and denial, the dam burst.

"You're right," Josie said to Chelsea. "I'm a woman." Her voice raised a little. "I'm a woman." She began to cry. *"I'm a woman!"* Josie described having an emotional breakdown right there in the bar. The anxiety of her life had prompted her to analyze the issue over and over, never resolving it. Then, during a time of distraction mixed with a pleasant mood, her friend hit her with an emotional appeal. There was an overwhelming feeling of rightness; there was no going back.

Because of bigotry, there was struggle, but Josie had passed through a one-way door. She began hormone therapy, saying, "There was a euphoria. You feel like your body chemistry is lining up with your brain for the first time." She legally changed her name and gender in early January 2017, hastening the process due to the election of Donald Trump. She feared it would prove difficult after he took office.

A few months later, she passed her registered-nursing exam and had her license issued in her new name. "It was a good feeling," Josie said. Now she has "a great job" in psychiatric nursing in Fargo, where she feels accepted.

"I am no longer living in denial in myriad ways. It goes way beyond gender presentation." She is free to express who she is and how she feels as a woman. "It's who I am now."

I once wrote an article for which I interviewed six different people who had been rejected by their families for their sexuality or gender identity. Much to her surprise, Josie said, that didn't happen to her. "They've come further than I ever imagined," Josie said of her parents. "It's not questioned anymore. It taught me a lesson that I shouldn't underestimate people's willingness to adapt."

Reinforcing the Magic Moment

Every day, Josie gets the positive reinforcement of knowing she's living the life she was meant to. It was a complete and total shift in identity—permitting her *true* self to finally reign—that forever changed her life.

This next part is some of the most interesting research in this book, and it's critical to the reason I wrote *The Holy Sh!t Moment,* because adherence always fascinated me. From my earliest days writing for the *Los Angeles Times,* I enjoyed examining what made people able to stick to certain regimens.

Adherence is everything.

Using weight-loss diets as an example, it's not whether you go south paleo, keto beach, veganomic, or full potato. When lowering the number on the scale is your goal, all that matters is your ability to sustain caloric restriction. Mind you, a higher *quality* diet is going to make it easier to reduce the *quantity* of calories consumed, but there are multiple methods for creating a quality, calorie-controlled diet. And study after study reveals the ability to stick to the diet is what is critical. Same goes for exercise; it could be the master class of building muscle and burning calories, but if you hate it and never go, it's useless to you.

To repeat, this is not a weight-loss book, unless you want it to be. Weight loss is just one of those examples for which "sticking to it" is most arduous.

But Chuck Gross stuck with it. As did Lesley, and me too. Regardless of the life change, there is a critical brain activity that keeps people on track post-epiphany.

It's the release of dopamine.

"It's a catastrophic phase change," said Colin DeYoung, a psychology professor who, appropriately, runs the DeYoung Personality Lab at the University of Minnesota.

Many people who had life-changing epiphanies tried the slow-and-steady behavior-change method, he explained, and they failed. "The slow method wasn't getting them anywhere." Agreeing with what Professor Ken Resnicow said, if the system, meaning your brain, is pushed in just the right way, "it leads to a spontaneous reorganization."

And when that happens, a lot of dopamine is released. Opioids too. The dopamine is about the excitement—the adventure of it all: you're about to embark on something good. The opioids are what make the event feel pleasurable.

Evolution programmed our brains to behave this way. This is not just a human thing. "Evolution doesn't have a particular start date," DeYoung said. This is a basic system because *all* organisms are goal oriented.

DeYoung had a study published in 2013 in *Frontiers in Human Neuroscience,* in which he referred to dopamine as "the neuromodulator of exploration."

Dopamine signals positive potential. When we encounter something unknown or unexpected, there is a dopamine reward response to this new information, the same way there is with more tangible rewards, such as consuming a tasty treat. "And what's going on with an epiphany or new insight is that it's a new piece of information, and you understand something you didn't before."

It's great in the moment of discovery. How does it keep driving you?

Dopamine is a teaching signal, DeYoung explained. If something is unfamiliar yet promising, you need to explore it. That's how organisms thrive: exploring that which is potentially risky but also has the possibility of great reward. "It's not just about learning what things are, but actually driving behavior in the moment to explore further."

A 2000 study published in *Psychological Science* revealed we're cautious of new phenomena, and rightly so. DeYoung said that pleasant warm glow our ancestors felt might have turned out to be a lava flow, so a little paranoia was good. But fear can fade. The study involved seventy-four undergraduate students at the University of Georgia. Unfamiliar stimuli were flashed on a screen, then their moods were evaluated. The more repeated the exposure to a stimulus, the more positive their moods. The fading of caution with exposure is evolutionarily adaptive, so long as nothing bad happens.

The neuromodulator is continuously updating the models in your mind of how you view the world regarding what is important, useful, and rewarding. Dopamine provides flexibility to change your understanding of the world.

Dopamine, in short, tells you what is valuable.

And it doesn't even have to be pleasurable, in the conventional sense. You don't need opioids to come along with it to compound the effect. Dopamine can facilitate motivational reinforcement and lead to habit-formation even for things that aren't pleasurable.

It is the *ongoing role* of dopamine that is a critical component of the holy-shit moment. What good is an epiphany if it doesn't keep driving you? "As long as they are putting in that work, they are going to continue having a dopaminergic response to the progress," DeYoung said. Focus on that word: "progress."

Progress.

Progress. Progress. Progress.

It's in your head now. You're welcome.

One way to think about dopamine, he explained, is to envision it responding to things when they are *a bit better* than they were before. The crucial way we achieve goals is looking for what is called "incentive reward." It's not the reward itself, but a cue that we are moving *toward* that reward.

In his book *The Power of Habit,* in the chapter on keystone habits, author Charles Duhigg referred to these as "small wins." And a 2011 spotlight in *Harvard Business Review* revealed how gratifying and motivating it is for people to *see* the progress they make chipping away at a goal. But the goal must be meaningful to the person doing the work.

If your epiphany is to go back to school to achieve a new degree or designation—and if this is something meaningful for you—when you go online to look at courses, there is a hit of dopamine. Then you register for courses. Dopamine hit. Buy books. More dopamine. Go to first class. Pay attention. Study. Take tests. Write papers. Caffeinate. More study. All a little hit of dopamine each time, pushing you toward that goal, letting you know you're on the correct path with a continual feeling of rightness; it motivated Lee Holland through ten years of advancing her education so she could make a difference in the world.

Marie Curie said, "I was taught that the way of progress was neither swift nor easy." Because of dopamine, each little, slow, difficult advancement pushed her forward. And gave her cancer, but that's not the point.

The point is that there *must* be progress. "If things are going poorly, there will be less dopamine," DeYoung said. "It's an adaptive response indicating the goal may be unattainable."

If Kathrine Switzer inspired you, and you have an epiphany about running a marathon but can barely go a mile, running that solitary mile is still rewarding. After a time, you can run a little farther, and that is additionally rewarding. And so on. And maybe after that marathon, there will be a quest for a faster one. Perhaps one day, I'll see you at the start line in Boston.

Professor DeYoung has a caution about doubt. If you don't believe the reward is in your grasp, you'll be more likely to seek something rewarding in the present. That's why your rational-analysis process needs to do what I wrote earlier about the expectancy-value approach to motivation: dream big, but achievably big. Implausible is fine, impossible is not.

And be prepared to be relentless in the face of adversity.

To illustrate this, Mark Beeman told me the story of cancer researcher Judah Folkman, who had an epiphany about why removal of a primary tumor can spark smaller metastases elsewhere in the body. The insight that "explained everything" came to him while attending a Rosh Hashanah ceremony at the Temple Israel in Boston in 1987. Being at prayer is the epitome of distraction; it didn't come to him in a lab.

His colleagues did not accept his conclusions.

"He had to fight for ten years against the establishment," Beeman told me. "For those ten years, he persisted, because he was so sure he was right."

And he was. Folkman's sudden insight and ongoing research led to the development of new treatments to inhibit the spread of numerous types of cancer.

Entrepreneurs starting a business often make little money for years, but because there is progress, even though it is small, there is dopamine. And so there is persistence. One day, perhaps they will be showering their loved ones with expensive gifts for having faith in them and supporting their dreams, dreams they pursued relentlessly because they were certain it was going to work out.

In 2017, the song "Feel It Still" by Portugal. The Man permeated the airwaves, garnering the band an instant and massive fan base. Few such fans knew that the two founding members from a small city in Alaska had been struggling to find success for thirteen years, and the song was from the band's *eighth* album. "Feel It Still" hit Top 10 in seventeen countries and won the band Best Pop Duo/Group Performance at the 60th Annual Grammy Awards. Gwen Stefani's band No Doubt is another example of musicians struggling for years in obscurity before finding massive success.

Such people stick with it in the face of adversity because they're inspired, determined, and confident. The slow but continual release of dopamine throughout this process keeps them focused, keeps them striving. Granted, such dreams don't always come to fruition, sometimes for reasons beyond one's control. Know when to cut your losses.

Not all the wins are small, not all the victories little. There are bigger bursts of dopamine to be had when you achieve a milestone moment; it reinvigorates the rightness of your course.

It had been a year since my first published piece, in a running magazine, earned me two hundred dollars. For six months, I'd been writing a twice-weekly column for AOL for modest pay. Regardless, the *Los Angeles Times* liked what they saw. Without even trying me out, they offered me a regular column. I haven't worked with the editor for years, but I remain close friends with the woman who gave me that break. (Hi, Rosie!) That was a big win.

Albert Einstein said conceiving relativity was "the happiest thought of my life." Judah Folkman referred to his sudden insight as "a very big high."

A 2010 study into the aha experience, published in *Current Directions in Psychological Science,* explained the "positive affect" comes from the "truth and confidence" it initiates, "even before systematically assessing the solution's veracity."

The big high and the feeling of rightness leave an impression. It's a massive rush of dopamine and opioids, followed by an ongoing neuromodulator IV drip into your brain to keep you on the path of progress.

It can put you in a state of *flow.*

"Flow" is a highly focused mental state, first described by Hungarian psychologist Mihaly Csikszentmihalyi as "a state of effortless concentration so deep that [people] lose their sense of time, of themselves, of their problems"—be it for their chosen career, studying, music, chess, sport, or some other enjoyable, meaningful experience. Regardless of age, culture, education, or activity type, anyone can experience flow, a universal human quality, when passionately engaged. It is the intense concentration itself that is rewarding.

My wife and kids make fun of how I tune out the world while writing. It happens because I'm passionate about my work.

One more brain science thing before we wrap this chapter up, because who doesn't like jazz?

Well, actually, I don't. I've never felt it, but some people do. When professional jazz musicians are improvising and they're in that state of flow, they're feeling it. In 2008, using fMRI technology, researchers from the National Institutes of Health examined six professional jazz piano players engaged in musical improvisation. Such a performance is highly individual. The musician draws from their own creative viewpoint. Two interesting things happen in the brain during such a performance.

First is the focal activation of the medial prefrontal cortex. According to the study, this part of the brain "plays a role in the neural instantiation of self, organizing internally motivated, self-generated, and stimulus-independent behaviors."

The other occurrence is the widespread *deactivation* of lateral portions of the prefrontal cortex. This is the part of the brain where "goal-directed behaviors are consciously monitored, evaluated and corrected." It also assesses if behavior conforms to social demands using conscious self-monitoring of the individual and the environment to ensure they fit in.

When you're absorbed in an activity and the house could burn down around you, that's your brain in a state of flow. The internally focused part of the mind lights up; the outside world gets shut off.

Sometimes it annoys family members, but it gets shit done.

Act Now!

- Pull out your phone or log on to your computer and schedule ten minutes per day for the next few days for distraction-free reflection. No screens or books or music. Find a comfortable, quiet place to sit and let your mind wander about anything and everything.
- Keep cramming new and interesting bits of information, thoughts, ideas, and experiences into your mind. Grow the box of your thoughts. Widen the tunnel of your vision. Synthesize it. Analyze how you feel about it.
- Imagine what it's like to make it *unsafely* to death. Think on the possibility of life being a thrill ride rather than a casual stroll.
- Work until you get stuck so the problem "sticks in your craw—and your brain." Then shower, go for a walk, watch a funny movie, sit back and relax, or take a nap.

5

THE ROCK-BOTTOM HYPOTHESIS:
THE POWER OF EPIPHANY TO BATTLE ADDICTION

Now is the winter of our discontent / made glorious summer . . .
—WILLIAM SHAKESPEARE

It was the 1988 Winter Olympic Games, and to my folly I believed I might outdrink a pair of Australians.

I arrived home long after midnight to an enthusiastic welcome from my standard poodle, upon whom I promptly threw up. He looked at me with consternation, wondering what he could have done to deserve such ignoble treatment. Then he began lapping up the portion of the vile substance that had landed on the floor, probably catching a buzz from it.

It was not my finest hour.

I've had some low points, but I've never seen anything I would call rock bottom. Even prior to my first epiphany, my life could have been much worse.

When some hit bottom, they grab a shovel and begin to dig. Life is a thunderstorm of Egyptian plague frogs, and they go in search of syphilitic scorpions to sleep with. Others don't go that far down the rabbit hole of self-destruction. You may not have sunk low at all; it doesn't mean there isn't benefit in reading this chapter. You don't have to strike magma prior to climbing out of the hole you've dug.

The music industry seems full of those who've hit a life-threatening low point. I've spoken to a few of them.

Staring Death in the Face

In 2009, while on tour in Eastern Europe, Nick Carter of the Backstreet Boys made the same mistake I did in 1988, except in his case it was Russians. "I was partying every night and really depressed," Nick told me. "I was trying to keep up with the local Russians in drinking games and I was feeling terrible."

After a lackluster stage performance, he saw a physician who read him the riot act. Carter had alcohol-induced cardiomyopathy, which was weakening his heart, and if he didn't change, the doctor said, he would die.

Carter was only twenty-eight years old.

"It was really life or death for me," he said. "I just completely went extreme in the other direction." He quit drinking and doing drugs, used exercise as a replacement, and lost sixty-five pounds.

"I wanted to fight for my life," Carter said of the sudden change. When looking at the possibility of an early death, he decided he didn't want it that way. I asked him to tell me why—

I'll stop doing that now.

Phil Collen, guitarist for Def Leppard, has a physique that could grace the cover of a fitness magazine. This despite almost six decades on the planet. It was his sudden renunciation of alcohol that led to him becoming so fit.

"I was drinking to excess, and I started blacking out and not remembering what happened," he told me. "I was doing really stupid things like driving and buying stuff and not remembering any of it." It continued to get worse, and he tried to cut down, but it was futile. What started off as the "odd glass of wine" became "shots of Jack" by the weekend.

His epiphany arrived in Paris, April 1987. He was leaving for India the next day and out celebrating his girlfriend's birthday. He was halfway through his first drink, a glass of champagne, and suddenly decided he was done. He pushed it away and said to her that he wasn't going to drink anymore. Ever.

He has remained true to that promise over three decades now.

"It wasn't fun anymore," Collen said. "It was very black or white. I knew I had to go this way or that way."

Professor William Miller, who has specialized in treatment of addictions for decades, refers to this as walking through a one-way door—you can't go back through.

There was no struggle. From the moment Collen decided to quit, he lacked any doubt. The only problem was boredom. Drinking had been his hobby. Eventually, he replaced it with exercise and achieved a level of fitness most can only dream of.

Brent Smith, lead singer for Shinedown, was addicted to cocaine, oxycodone, and alcohol. The cocaine kept his weight down, but when he quit that, he packed on seventy pounds. He still drank a lot.

On November 1, 2012, his girlfriend, Teresa, sat him down and said his lifestyle was "not going to work." His girlfriend's approach was to find him a personal trainer. He met with the trainer for the first time five days later. "I remember walking into that gym with a bit of a hangover," Brent said. "I was in really bad shape." He said he was in a death spiral and wanted to do it for Teresa and for his young son.

"I had an epiphany working out with my trainer that day, and I haven't had a drink since."

Smith embraced the fitness lifestyle as a replacement reward, which is a common theme. When people give up recreational drugs and alcohol, they often do well to engage in physical activity because of the newfound energy. Daniel Baldwin is another celebrity I've spoken to who found sobriety via being inspired to get fit.

Although *The Holy Sh!t Moment* is about a sudden transformation of identity and values that, as an example, make ceasing the use of addictive substances a fait accompli, it doesn't mean one should ignore the physiological benefits of using exercise as a tool to help one get over the hump of withdrawal. Ample research reveals the effectiveness of activity interventions for battling addiction. Most drug and alcohol rehabilitation programs use exercise as part of the recovery process.

The Burning Platform

The burning platform is an analogy for making a giant leap when you have no other choice.

It's a story told in *Switch,* by the Heath brothers, used to illustrate the imperative nature of corporate change when facing crisis.

In 1988, a gas leak triggered an explosion on the Piper Alpha oil platform in the North Sea. For many of the men, the choice was nightmarish: burn alive on a disintegrating platform or leap 175 feet into the sea, which was also on fire. In the disaster, 167 lost their lives and 61 survived, many by jumping. Chip and Dan Heath admit it's a "ridiculous business cliché" to use the burning-platform analogy to motivate employees to change. When it comes to battling addiction, however, it can be more appropriate than you know. There are those who are looking death in the eye, and they can't help but jump in another direction.

Fear of loss can motivate massive change, and anxiety primes the brain for sudden insight. If you're desperate enough, you may be ready for a quantum leap of motivation to change your situation.

Your task is to evaluate your negative behaviors. How stable is the platform? Is it a small flame or a raging inferno? How critical is the scenario?

A 2005 study of 659 problem drinkers published in *Addiction* found that those who quit because of a transformational experience (hitting rock bottom / spiritual awakening, etc.) had a much higher success rate than those who weighed pros and cons or who were encouraged by a third party to quit.

It is these intense experiences that prompt rapid change in the identity-value construct, which makes breaking bad habits far easier.

I know it's ironic, considering his fondness for drink, but it's been a while since I quoted Sir Winston.

"There is only one answer to defeat, and that is victory."

Determine the True Goal

"No one smokes to hurt their lungs. No one drinks to harm their liver."

Harvard psychologist Ellen Langer, author of *Mindfulness,* said this to me, explaining the need to make sense of a behavior from the perspective of the person engaged in it. With cigarettes, one may have been looking for a stimulant. With alcohol, the behavior may have arisen out of a desire to calm oneself. "You're not doing it for negative reasons," she said. Most important, negative behaviors can be replaced by achieving the desired sensation via more positive methods. That's why exercise is so often lauded as a therapy for addiction: the runner's high is real. You're not the tripping-balls and slurring-words kind of baked, but it does come with a sense of euphoria and enhanced well-being.

Langer is a fan of using mindfulness practices to find rationalization behind destructive behaviors and using that information to determine a compensatory substitution for the act.

A task: If there are unhealthy, negative behaviors you are engaged in, uncover what the true goal is. If you drink too much, why do you do it? Are you *really* trying to *Leaving Las Vegas* your liver? Or is it something else? Examine why you started and why you continue. What is the payoff? Figure that out and hold on to it. We'll be using that information for mindfulness practices in chapter 9.

Langer echoes the need for identity shift. "If you *really* stop smoking, you then see yourself as a *nonsmoker,* you're not pulled by it any longer. But if you consider yourself to be an *ex-smoker,* it means you're still desiring that cigarette." In her book, Langer writes of how drug counselors notice that people addicted to heroin report significantly fewer withdrawal symptoms if they do not consider themselves to be addicts.

The Best of Times

Professor Kennon Sheldon explained epiphany is less about being at rock bottom and more about it being the right time. "Most people reading that Joan Baez quote wouldn't have gotten as much out of it as you did," he said of my experience seeing "Action is the antidote to despair" in my college paper. A week earlier or a week later it might not have had any effect on me either, he added. "You were at a moment that was just right."

What creates such a moment?

Mark Beeman goes back to anxiety vs. a positive mood. The anxiety primes, and then, like Wag Dodge did when chased by fire, you become resigned and let go. That's when a life-changing epiphany is more prone to strike. But it doesn't have to be that low of a low point.

"He was a father who went to pick up his children at the library," William Miller told me of a man who was a smoker. "It was raining, and he was sitting at the curb waiting for them to come out." He searched through his pockets, the glove compartment, and even under the seat to look for cigarettes, but there weren't any. So he began to pull away from the curb to go buy cigarettes and spied his children in the rearview mirror. He said to himself, "I think I can get to the store and back before they get too wet."

At this part of the tale I burst out laughing. I can imagine his children standing there in the rain—like Cindy Lou Who seeing the Grinch steal her Christmas tree—watching their father drive away, thinking, *Why, Daddy? Why?*

"And in that moment, he stopped smoking." Miller finished the story: "He didn't want to be a man who would leave his children standing in the rain to chase after a drug." It was a sudden shift in identity and values, making quitting easy.

This story is in line with a study of 918 smokers and 996 ex-smokers published in the *British Medical Journal* in 2006, which looked at such "triggering" events leading to unplanned quitting attempts that were an "immediate renunciation of cigarettes." What's more, compared with those who used a planned attempt to quit, such triggered ones underwent a more complete transformation and were more likely to be successful.

In Miller's book *Quantum Change,* desperation was a common theme among those who went through significant change, particularly among people who had a more "mystical" epiphany, which we will examine further in the next chapter.

I will repeat a task here. Don't bum yourself out too bad, but consider your level of desperation. Understand that anxiety primes the brain for epiphany by generating your analysis and problem-solving mode. A stressful state narrows the focus—for now—by dwelling on what is wrong, searching for a resolution.

Take some time. Examine what's wrong. The hole need not be that deep, but if there is a hole, take a look around at the muddy bottom, the filth-coated sides, the dank stench of decay. How did you get there? Why did you dig it? How does this all make you feel, being trapped in it?

Consider what it would feel like to climb out.

Separate from Self-Loathing

A desperate situation may not be of your doing. I do not lay blame. This next part requires a content warning regarding childhood sexual abuse.

In 2017, I wrote a piece for the *Chicago Tribune* about sex abuse and weight gain, for which I interviewed Dr. Vincent Felitti. In the early 1980s, Dr. Felitti uncovered the connection between "adverse childhood experiences" (ACE) and a host of negative physical and mental health outcomes, obesity included. He spent decades surveying and following thousands of patients and publishing dozens of research studies to better understand the phenomenon.

One thing he told me stood out: "It is widely unrecognized that childhood sexual abuse is remarkably common." I didn't recognize it, either, until I requested interview subjects via Facebook. The response was overwhelming; the stories heartbreaking.

It's not just the rate of obesity that is affected by ACE, but depression, anxiety, autoimmune disorders, suicide, and addiction. And they're not small effects; they're orders of magnitude higher.

As I pointed out in chapter 1, self-compassion is key. The hole may have been dug for you before you reached adulthood. If you're not already engaged in it, professional therapy may be of benefit in dealing with the negative consequences.

Nothing in this book is about self-blame. If you need additional help, please seek it.

One benefit of a quantum change, William Miller writes, is that it can involve a "release from longstanding patterns of negative emotion." It can help release you from fear, anxiety, and depression. Core values shift; sometimes this involves forgiving others, and sometimes it's about forgiving yourself.

Hitting rock bottom is about reaching a "breaking point." There is a sudden transformation. Miller writes in *Quantum Change*: "Major change simply must occur because the person is unable or unwilling to continue in his or her present course." In a moment, identity is reorganized into something far more cohesive. For the person who reaches such a breaking point, there are often competing desires and interests. It is like multiple personality disorder in reverse. The pieces of identity are reordered. "The crisis is resolved by that person becoming someone new." Unlike the old one, the new identity is stable.

"Those things that hurt," Benjamin Franklin wrote, "instruct."

In 2004, researchers from the University of Warwick in England conducted a review of thirty-nine studies and found, in some cases, Nietzsche was right. It is possible for that which does not kill us to make us stronger. It is called "adversarial growth": struggling with adversity can prompt a person to a higher level of functioning.

But perhaps only in certain circumstances. A more recent study, published by Norwegian researchers in 2013, examined the concept of post-traumatic growth and found it incomplete. "Perceived growth" after significant trauma *is* associated with higher levels of life satisfaction, but it "does not seem to protect against impaired functioning in the aftermath of trauma." Granted, they were evaluating 197 survivors of the horrific 2011 Oslo bombing attack, an extreme event with a high likelihood of creating post-traumatic stress.

I am not one of those people who believes "everything happens for a reason." In fact, I hate that saying. If I were to suffer a terrible loss—perhaps the death of a loved one—and someone said that to me, I would be vexed.

Terrible things happen, and we are left to pick up the pieces. Sometimes these things present opportunities to grow. You are still traumatized, but not always paralyzed.

The Myriad Forms of Addiction

Considering my background, I'd be remiss were I to forgo the discussion of food addiction.

It has become fashionable to tout substances such as sugar as being addictive, and news stories have perpetuated a myth that sugar is much more addictive than cocaine, but a 2016 review of the research conducted at the University of Cambridge asserts there is "little evidence to support sugar addiction in humans." The reality is, no specific food meets the criteria for being addictive in the same way that drugs and alcohol are. However, in a 2014 article published in *Neuroscience & Biobehavioral Reviews,* the authors found that while specific foods or ingredients are not addictive, the act of eating *can be,* although such addictions are uncommon.

Insert stupid joke about turning tricks for Twix here.

Just because true food addiction is rare does *not* diminish the reality that many of us have endless access to highly palatable treat food that is difficult to resist. Many in the modern world can pick up the phone and have pizza, ice cream, and cheeseburgers at the door before the show they're watching is over. Every time we turn on the TV, view a website, gas up, drive down a main street, go through the grocery store checkout, or even attend a work meeting, we're assaulted with visual and olfactory stimuli for food designed to create sensory overload in the taste receptors of not just our tongues but also our brains.

Think of how the smell of cinnamon buns permeates the senses when you visit a mall. For a person struggling on a diet, it can be cruel and unusual punishment.

If treat food is available, most of us will want to shove it in our faces. It's rewarding, at least temporarily. When that piece of chocolate melts on your tongue, it provides a moment of comfort. It is *so compelling* that many health professionals consider it to have addictivelike properties; you can become *psychologically habituated* to overeating certain types of treat foods, and this can wreak havoc on both physiological and psychological health.

And so one outcome of an epiphany beneficial for weight loss is to become someone who no longer feels such compulsion, a person who no longer needs that comfort from food. Someone whose behavior suddenly shifts to come in line with their values, and who significantly lowers the priority of eating for reward or as a form of self-medication.

Such people have found their antidote to despair, and peanut butter chocolate Häagen-Dazs wasn't it. Which isn't to say enjoying the occasional indulgence of ice cream isn't an effective method of sticking to a healthy diet. I mean, have you *tried* that flavor? Knowing I can enjoy it in moderation helps me eat healthfully the rest of the time.

Knowing You're Done

"April 16, 1993, is tattooed on my leg," Todd Crandell said.

Prior to that day was thirteen years of "absolute misery." Todd had lost family, friends, jobs, and opportunities—all to addiction. It had been expected he would one day play in the NHL but he was expelled from school in his senior year for snorting cocaine on a hockey team bus. He went from being offered hockey scholarships to a drugged-out death spiral that involved consuming every mind-altering substance he could get his hands on.

Crandell's mother committed suicide due to her own addictions when Todd was only three. There are often battles being fought that we cannot see.

But everything changed on that spring day in Sylvania, Ohio. The beginning of this tale was told to him by others; he was way too wasted to remember it. Not just on alcohol, but cocaine, marijuana, and Xanax.

He'd been on a bender for three days. The night before he'd been at a Guns n' Roses concert, and he was drinking at a local bar in the morning. He went to drive home, got a flat, and had the car towed to an oil-change facility. "I called a friend to pick me up, and in the process, I took my pants down and pissed all over the manager's desk in his office." They called the police, and Crandell was arrested for his third DUI, blowing a 0.36.

That's 4.5 times the legal limit, and it was only midday.

After being let out of jail, Todd went to his grandmother's house and returned to drinking. As he finished another beer, a sharp, striking message entered his mind—it was a mystical epiphany, overwhelming both in power and simplicity: "You're done."

I asked him how it felt.

"'Relief' is the first word that comes to mind," he said. "Followed by 'motivated.'" He *knew*, in that moment, the horror was over. He also knew he was in a lot of trouble. "My life was in a complete shambles; I knew I'd have to go to jail." At the same time, Crandell had absolute certainty he would get through it. "It was a combination of excitement mixed with *Oh, God, I have a lot to clean up.*"

There was still withdrawal. "I considered the puking and sweating part of the healing process. I started moving my body to help get the crap out of my system." Todd said the withdrawal "sucked," but knew he'd never have to go through it again.

Another thing Todd said sucked was the thirty-three days in jail. "I knew I just had to do the time, then my life would go in a new direction."

One aspect of the new direction was a return to playing hockey after a decade-long absence. He worked hard for eighteen months and made it to the semipro league. This was followed by meeting the woman who would become his wife, getting a bachelor's degree, raising four children, and completing twenty-eight full-distance Ironman triathlons.

His oldest daughter was born five years to the day after he got sober. "It felt like a reminder of how well I was doing."

There was a second epiphany, eight years after the first.

"I had come back from doing Ironman New Zealand in 2001, and a local newspaper ran a story about my life." The response was overwhelming. Police who had arrested him in his previous life called to congratulate him. People he'd done drugs with called to say they couldn't believe he was alive. Realizing what a gift of a new life he'd been given, he found his purpose.

"That's when I started the nonprofit Racing for Recovery," Todd said. It's a fitness-promotion program to assist people battling substance abuse. The free program has an annual 5K foot race, but it also hosts Olympic-distance and half-Ironman triathlons in many other cities. Close to one hundred thousand people have been involved in the program since its inception.

Todd has a word of caution for those looking to exercise to battle addiction.

"Sometimes people get off drugs and then all they do is exercise," he said. "They're just obsessed with something else. If you're just running, and not learning and healing, you're missing the point."

Saying Goodbye to the Old Life

Phil Collen lost a dear friend.

Rock and roll is not known for promoting longevity. Jones, Hendrix, Joplin, Morrison, Cobain, Winehouse; they made the age of twenty-seven synonymous with tragic death by indulgence. Def Leppard has seen its share of such tragedy.

Steve Clark was Collen's co–lead guitarist in the band. They were close; they were drinking buddies. Other than playing in the band, they had alcohol in common. After Phil got sober, they began to drift apart. Steve kept going to the pub for recreation, Phil went to the gym and for runs. Four years later, in 1991, Clark died at the age of thirty from an overdose of alcohol and prescription painkillers. Collen was devastated at the loss.

Those who become sober, suddenly or not, will lose friends, but not necessarily to death.

If the only thing you have in common with certain people is the use of drugs and/or alcohol, they may not be supportive of your sobriety. With a shift in identity and values, you must also face the reality of potentially needing to find a new group of people to associate with.

With Todd Crandell's message of "You're done" came another command: "Go do something else."

It's not just about an ending, but a new beginning. A winter of discontent transformed into glorious summer. Shakespeare's quote, from *Richard III*, refers to a turning of the tide in the Wars of the Roses. It describes how things can go from sucking to spectacular when you win a crucial battle.

Bouncing back from rock bottom isn't just about ceasing bad behaviors, but finding good ones to replace them with. There will be newfound energy; put it to use.

Revel in your glorious summer.

Gain without Pain

While there is ample evidence of people turning their lives around after hitting rock bottom, recall the "good to great" examples from chapter 3. There is also the 2013 study of 605 people published in *The Journal of Positive Psychology* examining "post-ecstatic growth." The research found positive experiences can open one's eyes to "new opportunities, goals, roles, and values." This happens especially if the positive event involves inspiration, awe, or elevation.

That's what happened to Lee Holland. She was inspired by the ability she discovered within herself to help others because of that one phone call. She experienced what it was like to be elevated to a role in society by which she could truly make a positive difference in the lives of others.

It is important to make clear the study also determined that more hedonic experiences—feeling joyful and content—were likely to result in *less* growth. If things are peachy, we get complacent.

Whether you are at rock bottom, still digging, or crawling out, a sudden shift can change it all. Endeavor to understand the reasons behind the behaviors. Peel back those layers; expose the true self and your most closely held values and beliefs.

And your behaviors will no longer rule you; your identity and values will take command of your behavior, putting you on the path to a better life.

One more Churchill quote to end the chapter:

"We shall draw from the heart of suffering itself the means of inspiration and survival."

Act Now!

- Evaluate your negative behaviors and determine the stability of the platform. Are there flames? How large is the fire? Is the platform disintegrating? How critical is the dilemma you face? Have you reached a breaking point at which you *must* jump?
- Endeavor to discover the true reason behind negative behaviors. Is it a desire for stimulation or relaxation that has manifested in

an unhealthy behavior? What could such desires be replaced with that are healthier in nature?

- Ask how you would need to view your identity to ditch self-destructive behaviors. What kind of true self would need to come to the fore to create a dramatic transformation?
- Use the anxiety generated by pondering your dilemma to engage in analysis and problem-solving. Work the problem till you get stuck, then distract by engaging in mood-uplifting or relaxing behaviors. Be ready to recognize and act upon a sudden epiphany.
- Consider what you could do with the newfound energy by ceasing self-destructive behavior.

6

THE HAND OF GOD:
EXPLORING RELIGIOUS EPIPHANY

I find your lack of faith disturbing.
—DARTH VADER

Sometimes I am a whole lot of not smart.

It was a starry night. My son, who was thirteen at the time, occasionally freaked out the lone loon on Katherine Lake by returning its calls, a trick he'd learned from his grandfather. It had been a wet summer in British Columbia, and for once we were allowed a campfire on our annual vacation; there was no ban.

We were roasting fat, cheese-impregnated smokies on the fire. Oily goo popped and sizzled as it sweated out of the sausages and dropped onto the coals below. It takes patience, practice, and a steady hand to cook them over an open flame and not end up with a dog that's lukewarm on the inside, burnt on the surface.

Mine was near perfect. I grabbed a bun and—

"AHHH-Dammit-Arg-Shit-Ow-Shit-Shit-Shit!"

Rather than rely on branches as cooking implements, my wife had purchased telescopic cooking prongs. The handle was wood; the extendable prong, metal. As I went to pull my smokie off the prong, I grasped the hot metal and burned the end of my thumb but good.

I mean, *it really hurt!* Getting burned, especially on a sensitive fingertip, can ruin an otherwise lovely evening. Fortunately, my physician wife believes in Eagle Scout levels of medical preparedness; her first aid kit was so massive, a planeload of hemophiliacs might crash into the lake, and she could deal. She pulled out the kit, cleaned the burn, slathered it in pain-numbing ointment, and bandaged my thumb. Coupled with another beer or three, my pleasant night by the fire was saved.

Think of how much it hurts when you get the slightest burn. How long can you hold your hand to the flame? What would it take for you to not react to the pain?

Thích Quảng Đức showed no signs of feeling pain as he burned alive.

It's a harsh tale I'm about to tell. The point is to relay the power of religious belief to strengthen one's resolve.

On June 11, 1963, Đức, a Buddhist monk, entered a busy intersection in downtown Saigon to engage in an act of protest that would be seen around the world. A significant majority of the South Vietnamese population was Buddhist. The president, however, was part of the Catholic minority, and his government enacted numerous discriminatory policies against the Buddhist population.

Đức sat down on a cushion, assuming a meditative lotus position. Another monk poured a five-gallon can of gasoline over him. Đức rotated wooden prayer beads through his fingers and chanted; he struck a match.

Đức was engulfed in flames, but did not cry out, did not move.

Monks, nuns, passersby, even police, prostrated themselves before the burning monk. Cameras snapped photos. President John F. Kennedy said of one photo, which later won the Pulitzer Prize, "No news picture in history has generated so much emotion around the world."

Đức's faith gave him the strength of purpose to not only sacrifice his life for his cause, but to tolerate unimaginable pain without giving any indication of feeling his flesh burn. The power that belief can bestow to control one's mind and body can be amazing.

Churchill (him again) wrote in one of his autobiographies, "The idea that nothing is true except what we comprehend is silly." I will not opine on that which cannot be known. Whether it is divine intervention generating supernatural strength, or something more earthbound, is a matter of individual faith. Approximately 85 percent of the world's population, by varying degrees, has religion. Some go through the motions, others are most devout. Although I am not adherent, I lack the hubris to dismiss the beliefs of so many of my fellow humans.

A Sense of Divine Presence

"Any time you have a religious epiphany, and it's felt to be given by God, there is a sense of divine presence," James Kellenberger, professor emeritus of philosophy at California State University, Northridge, told me. Kellenberger is the author of several books on religion, including *Religious Epiphany Across Traditions and Cultures*, and there *are* myriad examples of epiphany among the various world religions.

Examples include the Feast of the Epiphany celebrating the revelation of Jesus as the incarnation of God. Moses saw a burning bush and was delivered the Ten Commandments. Saint Paul saw a light from heaven while on the road to Damascus and transformed from persecuting Christians to becoming a follower of Jesus.

It's important to note "religion" does not always mean "God." The Buddha achieved enlightenment under the Bodhi tree; it is believed the event allowed him to understand the nature of the universe and attain Nirvana, without involvement of a higher power.

Native America in the Modern World

It is common for Native Americans to engage in religious rituals to achieve insight. One such ritual is called Haŋblečeya—the vision quest.

To learn more, I spoke with Sandor Iron Rope, a full-blood Lakota Native American who has held a number of leadership roles in the Native American Church, including twice being chairperson for all North America.

"Haŋblečeya translates to 'crying throughout the night,'" Iron Rope said. It is a traditional ceremony conducted at a sacred site, usually chosen by a "spiritual intercessor." Often, the person undertaking the quest is a youth seeking understanding of what their role will be in the community upon entering adulthood.

The quest can last from two to four days, involving fasting and constant prayer while alone, to attain knowledge of oneself and the Great Spirit. "When you deplete the body of nutrients, your spiritual being is heightened," Iron Rope said. "Your mentality is in tune at a different level."

After achieving a vision, the seeker comes down from the sacred spot and goes into a sweat lodge with a spiritual intercessor to discuss the insight they received for help interpreting it. "After that, you have a small meal of traditional foods—pemmican and some corn and berry juice—to help bring you back."

I asked Iron Rope of the outcomes of these ceremonies, and he replied, "For the most part, it is a life-changing undertaking."

Haŋbleceya is not the only method of seeking insight used by Native Americans. Peyote—a psychoactive substance—is used in Native American Church ceremonies to assist in attaining visions for helping individuals and the community.

"Peyote is spiritually harvested from southern Texas," Iron Rope said. He spoke of how, if there is need for healing or insight, it will start off with a prayer in the homeland, followed by a pilgrimage to Texas where the peyote is grown. Then an offering is made. "There is always a prayer to obtain the medicine. Our way of life is a prayer."

Upon returning home, there is an explanation as to why members of the church have gathered; what type of understanding they seek, what solution they hope to uncover. That complete, they engage in an all-night ceremony. The amount of peyote consumed is individual, based on the practitioner's own experience with it. Sometimes tobacco is smoked as part of the ceremony.

"The medicine helps to be one with the elements," Iron Rope said. Together, there is praying and chanting toward the goal of understanding. "The fire does talk if you listen."

Beware imposters.

"Cultural appropriation is alive and well," Sandor Iron Rope said. It is unfortunately common for non-Natives, sometimes adopting Native-sounding names, to sell "vision quests" to anyone who can afford them as a vacation experience. And in the case of James Arthur Ray, the practice proved fatal for three participants in 2009 due to a combination of dehydration and heat stroke. Ray charged people ten thousand dollars each for his version of a vision quest in the Arizona desert. He was found guilty of felony negligent homicide and sentenced to two years in prison.

Standing Out from Ordinary Experience

In his book on religious epiphany, Kellenberger writes of a "high-relief epiphany," which "stand out against the background of ordinary experience." These are "awe-filled events so disruptive of the natural course of things . . . as to overwhelm any human who experiences them." They can be pyrotechnic and psychedelic, and the recipient can even be frightened by the supernatural display. They are a "wonder-filled and wrenching encounter."

Sometimes, Kellenberger told me, they lead to religious conversion, what he refers to as a "metanoia." Such was the case with the story of Saint Paul.

Beyond the biblical stories, religious epiphanies have made their mark upon history.

A World-Changing Phenomenon

William James wrote of religious belief bringing about extraordinary change, and that such change occurs regardless of whether God is real. If you believe, or do not, it doesn't affect the reality that religiously inspired people have influenced the course of world events.

Mohandas Gandhi had an epiphany about the use of the spinning wheel to engage people in an act of self-discipline that could commit his followers to large-scale collective action.

Martin Luther King, Jr., had an epiphany in the kitchen; he proclaimed Jesus spoke to him: "Martin Luther, stand up for righteousness. Stand up for justice. Stand up for truth. And lo, I will be with you, even until the end of the world."

During a grave illness, Mary Baker Eddy was reading the Bible and had a profound spiritual awakening that led to her founding Christian Science and launching an extensive literary output that would influence many women of her time and beyond.

Bill Wilson called out to God for help in battling his alcohol addiction, and in one form or another, he received it. This epiphany led to him co-founding Alcoholics Anonymous.

And one of the most impactful epiphanies of the last thousand years came from Martin Luther reading Ephesians 2:8–9, which states, "For by grace you have been saved through faith, and that not of yourselves; it is the gift of God, not of works, lest anyone should boast." Up until that time, Luther had been taught salvation was something one must *earn* via good deeds, but this reading generated a sudden awakening that salvation was achieved via faith, not labor. Thus began the Protestant Reformation.

And we must not forget that a mission from God prompted Jake and Elwood Blues to get the band back together and save the Saint Helen of the Blessed Shroud Orphanage.

What's Going On?

Miller and C'de Baca refer to the difference between an insightful epiphany and a mystical one as a bimodal distribution along a continuum. James Kellenberger, however, refers to it as more of a scatterplot distribution. There are myriad examples of epiphany, both religious and secular, that don't fit neatly along a straight line. Considering the overwhelming complexity of our brains and of the human experience, it makes sense there would be a phenomenal variety of phenomenal insight.

Our upbringing may have something to do with how insight manifests.

"If you're Jewish, it will be Jewish imagery. If you're Islamic, it will be Islamic imagery," Ken Resnicow said of religious epiphany. Same for Christian or any other religion. "The universe will talk to you through your spokesperson."

Mark Beeman discussed how many people use their religion to organize their thoughts and lives. If they cannot find meaning via secular methods, they often utilize religion. He said of life-changing epiphanies, "For some people it makes sense this would happen through a vision of

God or another aspect of their religion." On that note, Kellenberger said a religious epiphany didn't need to include God to qualify as one, just some form of presence, otherworldly or no.

"The right temporal lobe is where God touches you," Beeman said, referring to the part of the brain commonly called the "God spot"; it is activated during moments of intense religious belief—not exclusively activated, but considerably. Recall this is the same area of the brain primarily lit up during sudden insight. "It's another form of understanding about your life," he said, referring to the mental boxes we construct. If the box is focused on faith, then sudden insight can seem delivered by God.

It makes sense, except William Miller reported this was only sometimes the case. Often, recipients of a mystical epiphany are either not religious or only somewhat religious. A more common theme was for them to be in a state of desperation, perhaps hitting rock bottom.

From the people Miller and C'de Baca studied, one-third were praying at the time of their quantum change. Some of them had not prayed in years; for others, it was their first time ever. And prayer can take myriad forms. Some may view it more as meditation than appeal to a deity.

The researchers did notice there were unique aspects of mystical quantum change that didn't apply to a more insightful type of epiphany. The mystical variety is more about feelings than thoughts; there was a greater sense of significance and authority; it was something over which they did not have control—it happened *to* them, and there was a tremendous sense of awe. It may even involve an out-of-body sensation, like what happened to Josie Thomson with her near-death experience. It is also more common, compared to an insightful epiphany, for such recipients to recall specific details of the experience, including the time and date, long after it happened.

Imparting Great Strength

When my son was a toddler, he often refused to go to bed at night. To procure compliance, I chased him around the house, flinging water at him from a sippy cup, shouting, "The power of Christ compels you! The power of Christ compels you!"

But the power didn't flow. I couldn't compel shit. Same deal with his sister a couple of years later. Perhaps if it had been actual holy water . . .

Maybe it's divine, maybe it's dopamine. What is undeniable is that the recipient of a powerful religious epiphany, when given a mission, is *motivated*.

Kellenberger spoke of the historical examples listed previously. "They were people who became extraordinarily driven."

In terms of battling addiction, many have used faith to achieve sobriety. Being in a chemically altered state at the time, Todd Crandell didn't then realize it was a religious epiphany inspiring his sudden sobriety. But as he dwelt on it over the years, he came to feel the message arrived to him via both God and his mother's spirit. He said it has given him a faith he lacked prior to that day, although, "I mostly keep it to myself. I'm not out waving Bibles around."

Research suggests religious belief can be a powerful tool for overcoming drugs and alcohol. A 2007 study of 733 participants conducted by the Alcohol Research Group determined spiritual change during quitting attempts was "associated with significantly higher odds of abstinence at 12 months." And as reported in *Recent Developments in Alcoholism* (Springer, 2008), researchers at Duke University Medical Center found recovery from addiction is influenced through religious belief via "provision of a community, a narrative framework for meaning-making, a means of coping through submission and redemption." It could be more about the social aspect than belief in God, however.

It makes sense that, for someone who believes they have been commanded by a higher power to do a thing, they're going to be more inclined to do that thing.

In God's Hands

April Fool's Day 1996 was no laughing matter for country music star Clay Walker.

Walker has had six songs hit the number-one spot on the *Billboard* Hot Country Singles & Tracks chart. One of those songs, from 1993, is appropriately titled "Live Until I Die." Walker, who was only twenty-six at the time, and a new father to a baby girl, was about to be told he had eight years to live.

April 1 was the last show of the tour, in my hometown, Calgary, Canada. Prior to the concert, he was playing basketball with the band and began stumbling and falling. He laughed it off at first. Then there was double vision and facial spasms. His hands stopped working. He couldn't hold a guitar pick. He couldn't walk.

But the show must go on.

He was assisted to the microphone with the curtains drawn. The curtains opened, he sang, the curtains closed.

"I didn't move around that night," Clay told me. "I was terrified."

He returned home to Houston and went to St. Luke's Hospital. Over thirteen hours of tests later—MRI, blood work, a spinal tap—he had his diagnosis: multiple sclerosis.

"I asked the doctor what was going to happen, and he said I'd be in a wheelchair in four years and dead in eight. It was like driving a sword right through my body."

Clay was broken, his spirit wounded. He went home and held his baby girl close, and rather than saying, "Why me?" he asked, "Why now?" He couldn't sleep and cried through the night. Come morning, he put on his robe and walked to his home office, shutting the door.

Walker was not a devout man. Growing up, he had occasionally gone to church, but fell away from it in his teenage years. He had prayed on rare occasions, when he felt he needed something.

"I fell on my face and started to pray," he said. Walker describes what happened next not as prayer, but as having "a conversation with God." He asked God what he had planned for him. "If this is the end," he recalled speaking to God, "I accept it, but it's hard to believe you've brought me this far just to end it. Surely I can serve some other purpose."

Walker told me he heard God's reply with three simple words: "I have you."

An overwhelming sense of peace accompanied the words. In that moment, everything in Clay's life changed. He rose from the floor, picked up his guitar, and began to play—not his usual repertoire, but old hymns he knew. He played and he sang, feeling the power of the music and his belief flow through him. He walked out of the room a different man, sensing God would look after him no matter what happened next.

He went to see a specialist, telling his then wife whatever was to come, he could face it. Even if he was going to die, Clay Walker would be unafraid.

I am reminded of the words of Ralph Waldo Emerson: "God will not have his work made manifest by cowards."

Over the next year he had five more attacks, but he also became obsessed with learning everything he could about his condition. "What has turned my life around has been learning about MS, because we don't know that much," he said. "Had I not searched for that information, I'm not sure I'd be here today."

Walker told me how MS constricts the muscles, making you so tight you can't do normal exercises. Through a rigorous process he learned how to stretch through it, using the help of another person to push further than he could go on his own. It is the intense stretching regimen that allows him to stay active. "I can do pretty much any exercise another person can do, but I gotta get a lot of grease in the wheels before I start rolling."

A big part of his life revolves around fitness to keep his condition at bay. One thing he does on tour is tow a trailer full of bicycles behind the tour bus. "Me and my band will ride 25 to 40 miles a day. People with MS have their timing messed up, because their legs don't work in sync. Riding a bike really helps me sync them."

Clay spoke of how the intense stretching and exercise, medication, and focusing on a healthy diet has allowed him to reclaim what he lost from MS and stop the attacks.

For the next fifteen years he had the same neurologist, Dr. Jerry Wolinsky. On a whim, while sitting in a hotel room in Los Angeles, he called Dr. Wolinsky to ask him a question. He told him of the initial prognosis from a different doctor: he'd be in a wheelchair in four years and dead in eight. Wolinsky replied, "That would have been my same prognosis for you."

Five years later, Dr. Wolinsky was retiring and handing Clay's case over to a colleague, Dr. John Lincoln. As part of the process, Lincoln had to examine Walker's records from the past two decades and do his own medical workup on Clay. After completing the process, Lincoln and Wolinsky were chatting about Walker, with him in the room.

"It's a miracle," Lincoln said of Walker's condition. Clay asked what he meant by that, and the doctor replied, "It's very rare to see someone with your amount of lesions on the brain stem and spinal cord, and not have the disease progress." Clay asked him how often he'd seen that happen, and Dr. Lincoln said, "Never."

"That moment in 1996 was a turning point," Clay Walker said, of hearing the voice of God. Those three simple words, "I have you," infused him with courage and an abiding faith that changed the path of his life and his illness. "I'm very religious now," he said. "I'm deeply Catholic."

Alas, prayer doesn't work for everyone. Many are desperate and send out an appeal, but inspiration doesn't arrive. Walker is an example of "Results not typical."

Now the father of six children, Walker continues to compose and perform music. Shortly before our conversation, he sang the National Anthem to open Game 5 of the 2017 World Series. In 2015, his family built a new house and intended to have a small recording studio on the property, but he decided to turn the building into a chapel instead. "It only holds about ten people. I go in there and pray every day for a few minutes."

Walker is appreciative of the variety of world religions, saying they are filled with people with honest hearts seeking a relationship with God. The morning of April 3, 1996, was the day Clay Walker forged that bond.

"For me, in that moment, it became so real. It changed everything for me."

The Neutral Observer

Clay Walker's experience is an inspiring tale his fellow faithful will feel an emotional connection to. Others may be skeptical regarding the nature of the lack of disease progression or the voice he heard. What is undeniable is that he was inspired to battle his condition via a demanding regimen.

People have these experiences. The experiences are profound. Such events change lives by motivating the recipient to action.

James Kellenberger spoke of the neutral observer to such a phenomenon, using the epiphany of Saint Paul as an example. "The observer can explain his conversion experience without any reference to a divine incursion," he said. Someone could have knowledge of the man's history, that he was known as Saul of Tarsus, a Roman citizen from a devout Jewish family. He was dedicated to the persecution of the early followers of Jesus. And then, sometime around the age of thirty, Saul was traveling to Damascus and saw a flash of light. This light could have been any variety of natural phenomena. Saul fell to his knees and was heard to cry out, as you might expect of a man who had been struck blind by a bright light.

Saul had to be led into Damascus by hand and did not regain his sight for three days. Afterward, he changed from persecuting the followers of Jesus to becoming a devoted believer in his teachings and a leader in the Christian ministry.

As you can see, you can tell that tale of what appeared to happen without referring to anything supernatural. It could have been a meteor flash that blinded Saul. But, Kellenberger explains, when you tell the story from the perspective of Saint Paul, the reference to the divine must be included, because that is what he experienced. "It's a matter of perspective," Kellenberger told me. "For Clay Walker, there is a felt sense of the religious wrapped up in a seemingly miraculous event. When that happens, how one is affected can be extraordinary." It creates a sense of awe and wonder and reverence before God.

This is the only task I'll present for this chapter, and, due to the nature of the subject matter, it's up to you how or even if you follow it.

You may have minimal or perhaps significant belief. Alternatively, you may have none. Regardless, consider two things:

1. Prayer can result in a massive change in a person, even if a higher power does not exist.
2. From Miller and C'de Baca's research, approximately one-third of those who experienced a life-changing epiphany were engaged in prayer at the time. "It was the single most common act preceding quantum change," the authors wrote. What's more, for

many such people, they had either never prayed before or it was their first prayer in a long time.

And so, taking those two realities into consideration, I ask you to think about the use of prayer for helping achieve a life-changing insight. Especially if you are in desperate circumstances. It doesn't have to be prayer, per se. It can be a meditative activity that creates sudden comprehension to resolve a problem. On the same page of Churchill's autobiography where he wrote the previous quotation offered in this chapter, he also wrote that *how* we receive such messages matters not. Rather, "What is important is the message and the benefits to you of receiving it."

"One of the Bravest Persons Alive"

The 2016 film *Hacksaw Ridge,* which was nominated for six Academy Awards, including Best Picture and Best Actor, is the story of World War II conscientious objector Desmond Doss. Although Doss preferred to be referred to as a "conscientious cooperator."

Doss was awarded the Medal of Honor for his heroic actions during the battle for Okinawa in 1945—the bloodiest battle of the Pacific theater—despite his refusal to touch a weapon. Desmond Doss is an example of how someone can be religiously inspired yet have a life-changing epiphany delivered by insight rather than be mystical in origin.

Doss's mother was a Seventh-day Adventist and instilled the Ten Commandments in her children. I spoke with Desmond's only child, Desmond Thomas Doss, Jr. ("Tommy"), who grew up hearing his father's story over and over. We began our conversation discussing a picture that hung on the wall of his father's childhood home in Lynchburg, Virginia.

"It depicted the Ten Commandments," Tommy told me. "Each commandment had a little drawing, and the sixth said, 'Thou Shalt Not Kill,' and it showed a picture of Cain after he killed his brother Abel. He would gaze at it again and again. He had an obsession about that."

"He had this big club that he killed his brother with," Desmond Doss, Sr., said in the 2003 documentary on his life, *The Conscientious Objector*. "I wondered how in the world could a big brother do such a thing."

Doss's best friend was his brother Harold.

A defining moment that would set the course for the rest of Desmond Doss's life arrived when the image of Cain killing Abel almost became real before his eyes. His father, William Thomas Doss, was a decorated veteran of the First World War who suffered PTSD. It was the Great Depression, and the man turned to drink as a way to cope. "It's an experience I won't ever forget," said Desmond Sr. of one fateful night. "My uncle and my dad were both drinking . . . and they got into a fight."

Insults were thrown, challenges issued. In the heat of the moment, Desmond's father pulled out a .45 caliber pistol. "Mother got in between, and neither one of them wanted to hit mother," Desmond said. "And mother told them, 'You give me that gun!'" She took the gun and handed it to Desmond, who was only a boy, and said, "Go hide that gun!"

Desmond took the gun and ran.

The pistol safely hidden, he ran back to see the police hauling his father away in handcuffs. "I'll never forget that experience, because if it hadn't been for my mother, my daddy most likely would have killed him." The image of Cain killing Abel above the words "Thou Shalt Not Kill" burned into Desmond Doss's mind, he swore it was the last time he would ever touch a gun.

That vow would not come without consequences. Nevertheless, he remained resolute.

In 1942, with war ravaging the world, Doss registered for the draft and was called up. Working at the Newport News Naval Shipyard, he qualified for a deferment but wanted to do his part. "I felt like it was an honor to serve God and country." His desire was not to take lives, but to save them.

He was classified as a conscientious objector, a designation he didn't want. "When I told the sergeant I was supposed to be a medic, he said, 'We tell you what to do. You don't tell us nothing.'" The army tried to break him. Despite his designation, they assigned him to a rifle company, refusing his request to be a medic. Doss was abused by his fellow soldiers and given the worst duties by his superiors. They tried to get him to quit, to get him sent to a conscientious objector camp, even to have him declared mentally unfit.

"One fella, he told me, 'I swear to God, Doss, you go into combat, I'm gonna shoot you,'" Desmond said of one of the men in his unit. When he refused to even touch a rifle during training, he was threatened with court-martial. According to his biography, *Redemption at Hacksaw Ridge,* he respected his superiors, but "he had received a prior order from a Higher Authority. . . . He did not consider the Ten Commandments as mere guides." Realizing Doss was steadfast, after a month they transferred him to the medical corps.

Doss was awarded the Bronze Star for valor twice, for his actions on Guam and Leyte. The story of his superhuman heroics, which won him the Medal of Honor—the highest U.S. military honor—is the stuff of legend. In fact, the movie *Hacksaw Ridge,* which is an accurate portrayal of Doss's bravery, left out certain parts of Doss's tale because they were deemed too unbelievable for the film.

In May of 1945, despite suffering from tuberculosis, Doss was with the Ninety-Sixth Division as they attempted to take the Maeda Escarpment, nicknamed "Hacksaw Ridge," on Okinawa. After a vicious counterattack by the occupying Japanese forces, the Americans retreated back down a sheer cliff using cargo nets. Less than one-third of the men made it back down.

Desmond Doss stayed behind.

Through the rest of that day and night, at constant risk of death from patrolling Japanese soldiers, Desmond Doss searched for his wounded comrades who were left for dead. He treated their wounds, dragged or carried them to the edge of the cliff, and fashioned a rope harness to lower them down the escarpment to safety.

With no weapon to protect himself, more than seventy-five times he repeated this action.

When the American forces went back up to take the ridge, Doss was with them. He was severely wounded in that action but survived and lived to be eighty-seven.

One of the many lives Desmond Doss saved was that of his captain, Jack Glover, who had tried to get him transferred to a conscientious objector camp during training. Glover later said of Doss, "He was one of the bravest persons alive."

God Leaves the Building

Things don't always work out the way they did for Clay Walker or Todd Crandell. In some cases, rather than experiencing the metanoia of religious conversion, or being inspired to eschew violence, like Desmond Doss, people move in a different direction.

Jennifer Brown lives in Barstow, California, a small town halfway between Las Vegas and Los Angeles. She was raised just outside Dallas and attended a fundamentalist Baptist church. Brown described the church she attended as "an extremely hard form of Christianity, one step above snake handling."

Jennifer was an excellent student; a member of the National Honor Society, which required volunteer work. And so, she worked as a candy striper at the local hospital. She was sent to the pediatrics wing and got off on the wrong floor, the one for patients with HIV and AIDS. "The nurse saw I had the volunteer tag and said, 'You don't want to be here. This is a rough place.'"

Jennifer took her word for it and returned to the elevator, then decided, no, if these people were sick, she was needed. "I turned around and told the nurse, 'Give me what you got.'"

The year was 1997; Jennifer had just turned seventeen.

During her volunteering, she became close friends with David, a thirty-two-year-old gay man who was dying of AIDS. Her church had learned of her volunteer work and counseled Jennifer repeatedly on how she was to preach to David to get him to admit his sins, admit being gay was wrong, and that if he would decide to not be gay anymore and accept Jesus, he could go to heaven.

I asked Jennifer if she did any of that. "Hell, no!" was her reply.

Six months after meeting her, David succumbed to his illness. Jennifer had grown close to him and was devastated. She attended his funeral on a Friday, and the following Sunday she was in church; it was the day her life changed.

Prior to this, Jennifer was a dedicated believer. When she was troubled, she would sit in church, read her Bible, and find the answers to her problems. Church was a comforting presence in her life.

But two days after David's funeral, Jennifer was pulled out of the teen Sunday school by the pastor's wife and led to the church kitchen. In the room were several of the deacon's wives. They made her a cup of tea. Jennifer expected they knew she was upset about the loss of her friend and were going to console her.

That is not what happened.

"It launched into 'That lifestyle is wrong,'" Jennifer said. "'You have to believe in Jesus and not be gay,' they told me." According to these women, she wasn't supposed to be associating with *that community*.

The more they talked, the greater disconnect Jennifer felt. She described it as the air being sucked from the room. She got cold chills; she shivered and her teeth chattered. Any comfort she had felt from her faith evaporated in an instant.

Jennifer looked down at her teacup and was surprised to see it was empty. "In that moment, God left the building. I have never felt God since that day."

The loss of that sense of comfort and community had a negative effect on Jennifer for a time. She described slipping into typical teenage nihilism: "We're all going to die, and nothing matters."

But the loss of faith changed the course of her life. She had been instructed by her family and her church how her life was going to go: she was to attend a small Baptist college, learn to become a secretary, meet a man, and become a wife and mother.

"David had told me I was meant for much more than that," she said. "He told me I needed to go to a big college and major in something important to me." And so she rebelled against the desires of her family and her church and attended the University of North Carolina at Chapel Hill, receiving a degree in medieval history. For a time, she worked in museums, until she met her husband in 2009 and became pregnant the following year. She considers it ironic that she rebelled against being a stay-at-home mom and yet now is one.

But she still uses her college education. Her husband works as a Department of Defense contractor at Fort Irwin, which is why they live in what Jennifer describes as "the middle of nowhere." They have two children now; both are intellectually gifted. The local school is too small to provide an education that would allow them to flourish. Jennifer decided to homeschool them. "Secular homeschool, of course," she said. "There is no Jesus in class."

I asked her if the epiphany of losing her religion was a positive outcome. "I am glad it happened," she said. "It forced me out of my little box of what I thought I knew. Before, I would not have dreamed of going to college that far from home."

"There are epiphanies of all sorts," James Kellenberger said. "Not all amount to metanoia." In the case of Jennifer Brown, it was the exact opposite. Rather than a sensation of presence, it was the sudden fleeing of it.

The purpose of telling Jennifer's tale? Embrace the real self and you'll be okay. She wasn't destined to continue on that path. Whether God comes in or leaves, you must find *your* profound truth that allows your real self to come forward and thrive.

It's different for each person. Find the right path. Then walk it.

Act Now!

- Remember what I wrote about prayer. If you are reluctant, consider that God does not have to exist for it to be effective in inspiring change. Recall it was the most common act preceding epiphany in the study by Miller and C'de Baca. Contemplate if it is something that may help you. And, if it feels right, give it a try.

THE POWER OF LOVE:
HOW PASSION FOR LIFE AND LOVE
INSPIRES SUDDEN CHANGE

If there are no dogs in heaven, then when I die
I want to go where they went.

—WILL ROGERS

I mentioned throwing up on my poodle.

He was a big white one; friendly and smart. He loved to play tug-of-war with his blanket. I taught him to jump through a hoop. One time, when my mother was windsurfing, he ran up and down the beach barking at her because he could not conceive of what she was doing. He decided to swim out to her to ascertain what was up, then climbed onto the front of the board. They were a spectacle as they sailed along the shore, my dog's tongue lolling to the side, a thrilled look on his face like he was sticking his head out a car window.

Good times. When he died, I cried for days.

My sister had a standard poodle as well, a black female. The two dogs were tight. My mother loved them as well, and when they went on to dog heaven, she had them cremated and put into urns, placing them on the mantle side by side.

Years later, we were having a Sunday dinner at my parents' house, and I said I was tired of this morbid doggy-ashes-on-the-mantel stuff. I wanted to spread them.

If you've seen the movie *Brokeback Mountain,* there is a scene in which naked Jake and also naked Heath jump off a high cliff into freezing cold water. I've jumped off that exact cliff many times, as it's less than an hour's drive from my house. I'd taken the dogs there often (they didn't jump), and it was always an adventure. I told my mother I would spread them near the cliffs; she agreed.

At the time, my car was an Acura Integra hatchback. The divider that separated the back seat from the trunk had a broken latch that rattled, so I removed it. The dogs were in ceramic urns in the trunk. During the drive, a car in front of me slammed on the brakes for no discernible reason; I had to hit mine as well to avoid a collision.

The urns smashed into each other and broke. The ashes of our beloved pets filled the car. I inhaled some.

I pulled over, popped the trunk, and a portion of the two dogs wafted away across the countryside. I had a garbage bag full of books to donate residing in the trunk, and I repurposed the bag to carry doggy ashes, scooping them in with my bare hands as best I could.

I drove the rest of the way to the cliffs with the windows open to air out the car.

Once there, I spread *most* of our dogs' ashes around some trees at the top of a hill overlooking the river below. Before returning home, I stopped at a gas station to use a coin-operated vacuum cleaner to suck up the remainder of the dear departed doggies.

My mother is going to kill me when she reads this.

Love is powerful. It can prompt an ordinary human to extraordinary acts. And it need not be love of a fellow person to do so.

Looking on the Brightest Side

"When I look at the world, I'm pessimistic, but when I look at people, I am optimistic."

Carl Rogers married his high school sweetheart, Helen Elliott, in 1924, and they stayed together, raising two children, until her death fifty-five years later.

He believed in love.

In cooperation with Abraham Maslow, Rogers developed humanistic psychology, which values free will, creativity, and human potential. Rogers did much to achieve his own personal potential, dedicating the final decade of his life working toward world peace. Rogers was nominated for the Nobel Peace Prize the year he died, 1987.

He developed the concept "unconditional positive regard," which is about having compassion for your fellow humans, acknowledging their best potential. It is an attitude of grace, in which we value ourselves and others despite knowing our failings. It permits people to drop pretenses and open themselves to a full range of emotional experiences.

Problems arise when we feel defensive. The world and the people in it don't always go the way we want, and internal conflict arises between our ideas and external stimulus; we try to block it out or reinterpret reality so we don't have to challenge preconceived notions. The problem then becomes one of shutting off potential emotional reaction as wrong or inappropriate.

This doesn't mean you should do what you feel like all the time. If that were the case, I might never wear pants.

The idea is to be open to new, deeper, richer emotional experiences in every aspect of life. It may seem a challenge to be willing to acknowledge the positive potential of the person who just cut you off in traffic, but consider the work of Holocaust survivor Viktor Frankl before writing off that guy in the BMW who never uses his signal light.

An Austrian neurologist and psychiatrist, Frankl was the author of *Man's Search for Meaning*. In it, he writes of how the *striving* for meaning is the most motivating force in humans. What does that have to do with positive regard? Frankl draws parallels between our ability to feel love and find meaning in life.

"Love is the only way to grasp another human being in the innermost core of his personality," Frankl writes. To comprehend the essence of others, we must love them, and by doing so we are enabled to understand their traits and features, and, most important, their potential. We gain the ability to make them aware of what they can become, and they may do the same for us. It is mutually beneficial and, according to Frankl, the key to unlocking human potential.

This from a man who witnessed firsthand the worst of humanity during the Second World War.

Speaking of which, recall the story of Desmond Doss from the previous chapter. His son, Tommy, was adamant it was not his father's religious belief that prompted his remarkable bravery that saved the lives of so many on Okinawa in 1945. "There is not a preacher in the world who could do what my father did," he said. Rather, "It was his capacity for love that he developed in early childhood. He had a very loving mother. He loved his siblings, his church, his wife. He loved the men he served with and cared for." Doss Jr. explained he was pleased to see that the movie *Hacksaw Ridge* showed the part of his father's story in which he gave medical aid to a wounded Japanese soldier. "He had this unconditional love for people no matter who it was."

The Time Tunnel of Love

Baby, I love you so much I'd travel through time for you.

I'm pretty sure Keanu Reeves said that. Or was it Hugh Jackman? Eric Bana? Colin Farrell? I could go on, but instead I'll ask: How come it is usually the men in these romantic tales who are surfing the space-time continuum? Is it the whole "bad boy" thing? Like, "Hey, darlin', I just violated the physical laws of the universe. Now watch me ride a Harley while smoking a Marlborough and not wearing a helmet."

I do have a point.

That point is, we are all traveling through time, at a rate of one second per second. As of writing, I have spent almost nine hundred million seconds in love with my wife. She is my fellow time traveler.

I was about twenty-five million seconds into our relationship and concerned over not being able to spend a couple billion more with her, when my life-changing epiphany struck. As it turns out, such long-term thinking has the power to trigger insight, whereas focusing on the short-term constricts it.

A 2004 study published in the *Journal of Personality and Social Psychology* conducted six experiments to test analytic vs. creative ability. When the participants imagined working on an insight problem a year in the future, they were more successful than those told to imagine working on it the next day. The long-term thinkers also found it less challenging to arrive at the solution.

What does this have to do with love?

Five years later, the same lead researcher from the previous study, Jens Förster, out of the University of Amsterdam, examined how sex and love influence creative vs. analytical thinking.

The stuff people get paid to research . . .

In the first study, researchers either "love-primed" or "lust-primed" the participants. They devised a way of doing so while keeping everyone's clothes on, FYI. The love-primed were asked to imagine a long walk with their partner and to ponder how much in love they were. If they didn't have a partner, they were asked to imagine an ideal person to fall in love with. (On an unrelated note, I've interviewed Hugh Jackman, and he's just as wonderful as you imagine.) The lust-primed were asked to imagine a casual sex scenario with someone they were attracted to but not in love with.

Guess who was better at insight and who was better at analysis.

Lust-priming made people *suck* at creativity. How do we know? The control group did *three times* better at solving creative insight problems than the lust-primed. And the love-primed did more than five times better. This might explain why pickup lines are usually so shitty. With so much focus on blood flow to the nethers, the creative brain gets shut off.

But the lusty kicked ass at analytical problems: they were much better than the control group and performed almost twice as well as the love-primed group. I expect that's good for going through checklists of things, like having birth control and figuring out what remote location is best to park the Chevy in.

The researchers conducted a second study using priming words such as "love," "loving," and "to love," vs. "sex," "eroticism," and "sexuality." The results weren't quite as dramatic, but there was still far superior creative processing in the love-primed, and better analytical performance in the lust-primed.

The researchers put it down to long-term vs. short-term thinking, but Kounios and Beeman wrote of the study in *The Eureka Factor,* offering further opinion on the outcomes. Being in love is surmised to create greater happiness than being lusty, and positive mood helps foster insight. What's more, people who are in love need to consider the perspective of their partners: their likes and dislikes, and what they wish for the future. Love creates a demand for cognitive flexibility to think outside our own mental box.

Lust, conversely, is a little more constricted to *How do I get this person to want to take their clothes off in private with me?*

Let's make a task of this, shall we? No need for privacy. You can stay dressed.

If you're in a relationship—a good one, I mean—consider your love for that person. Think about your future together and how your hopes and dreams merge with theirs. Ponder something ideal, then apply those desires to what needs to happen today to bring it to fruition.

While you're at it, contemplate giving unconditional positive regard a try. In every long-term relationship, we will discover things about a partner that drive us bugshit. Understand you have habits that make them equally bonkers. Choose to see them as their best possible selves.

A Path to Knowing

"Love is a bridge . . . from poorer to richer knowledge." These are the words of German philosopher Max Scheler in his 1923 essay "Love and Knowledge." He referred to love as "a kind of spiritual midwife" by which self-knowledge is gained.

Cogito ergo sum is a Latin proposition by seventeenth-century French philosopher René Descartes. In his 1637 work *Discourse on the Method* (truncated), Descartes translated it to "I am thinking, therefore I exist." Most will know it as, "I think, therefore I am."

Max Scheler would disagree. To be fully human is not just to be someone who thinks, but a being who loves. That is because we achieve who we are not via just rational analysis, but through how we feel. Rider and elephant. Cognition and emotion. System 1 and System 2. All that stuff.

But one must be wary not to sacrifice too much of the self in the acceptance of another.

Balancing the Needs of Others

Be cautious of "pathological altruism," Scott Kaufman warns. It's when we put the needs of others so much in front of ourselves we cause self-harm. It can lead to depression and burnout when we give too much of ourselves. Kaufman mentioned that eating disorders are common in those who engage in pathological altruism. "It is a form of self-hate," he said. "It's maladaptive."

Consider this a warning that life is not all about self-sacrifice. You need to be getting something positive out of your relationships.

"Susan" wasn't.

She'd been with a man for four and a half years. Susan was willing to use her full name, but I changed it to protect her ex's identity; you'll soon understand why. The first year and a half were good, but they hadn't had sex in three years. "We were more like roommates, but I still cared about him," she said. A year into the relationship she moved from Illinois to Florida with him, so he could attend school. Susan paid for everything.

The man had a history of drug abuse but had been clean for three years before they met. Four years into the relationship, in 2016, she was shocked to find him not breathing, his skin blue. "I called 911 and watched them give him NARCAN," Susan said. "I was really scared." To this day, when she hears an ambulance, she has flashbacks to that moment. She needed therapy for the trauma of seeing the man she loved almost die from an overdose.

"The relationship had been awful for the prior two and a half years," but her initial reaction to the overdose was loving. "I really wanted to help him. I was positive things would get better." But they didn't. His drug of choice was oxycodone, but she also discovered he'd been buying heroin from prostitutes. "He was spending eight hundred dollars a month on drugs." In

2017, six months after the first overdose, her boyfriend did it again. In the hospital, she realized she was embarrassed to be this man's partner, to be supporting him in his self-destruction. "I had tried really hard for six months, and he'd been lying to me," she said. "In that moment, I realized I had no love left for him, and I had to get out."

The next day, at the age of thirty-two, she applied for a job transfer to California, where her brother lived. She had to give thirty days' notice at her current position, and during that time her now ex-boyfriend "used a lot of guilt and blame and crying, asking me to stay, but my mind was completely made up."

And now? "I have an amazing life. I love where I live. I'm making friends and dating an amazing man."

Gloria Steinem said, "Far too many people are looking for the right person, instead of trying to be the right person."

"It comes from a place of low self-worth," Kaufman told me. The opposite of low self-worth is self-acceptance, and people who accept themselves are more in tune with who they are; it's valuable for attaining life-changing insights. "They don't feel like they're wearing a mask all the time." They are more authentic—something Carl Rogers encouraged—and they are more trusting of their intuition and emotions. This is why it is important to be in relationships that increase your self-worth, not lower it.

A task: If there are relationships that, deep down, you know you need to reevaluate, do it. It won't be easy. Do it anyway.

And if it leads to an ending, please leave my name out of it. I don't want any angry exes knocking on my door.

Filling the Tank, Not Draining It

I told you about my meeting The One, and how fear of losing her prompted a life-changing epiphany. That is one example of how love can inspire sudden and massive change.

My website is bodyforwife.com.

It was a joke among friends from when the *Body for Life* book was popular. I like that she appreciates my efforts, but I mostly pursue fitness for me.

Nevertheless, there are many things I do for my wife, sometimes when I'd rather not. Sometimes they become like a duty, but a relationship is multifaceted. John Lennon was wrong. Love is not all you need.

In a relationship, you don't just get to do what you feel like. Taking a note from Carl Rogers, I look at her with unconditional positive regard and see she is often doing things she'd rather not that benefit me.

I do her laundry, she does my taxes. I do the cooking, she manages our finances. I work hard to please her, and my tank is full. This is how it should be. Life is not a zero-sum game. For one to win does not mean another must lose, and vice versa. My wife has accomplished great things with my support, and she has returned that when I needed it. I would not be who I am today without her.

She's my muse. She's brilliant and hardworking and kind. She has faced arduous trials in life and come through like a champion. She inspires me with that "You make me want to be a better man" kind of stuff. Apparently, I inspire her as well.

Love makes us stronger. United, we stand.

Even when I was catching kid vomit in my bare hands, there was a payoff. And I'm not just talking about less to clean up from the carpet. Toddler meltdowns can be epic, but snuggles and "I love you, Daddy" are worth it. To me, they are, because my real self wanted children. Not everyone should be a parent, however.

Love can prompt us to be our best selves; it can start before the object of that love enters the world.

A Teachable Moment

"Pregnancy is a time in your life that is a teachable moment," said Benjamin Gardner, a senior lecturer in psychology at King's College London and an expert in habit formation.

We spoke of "the behaviour change wheel," a framework on which all behavior is a combination of capability, motivation, and opportunity. "Anything that changes behavior has to change one of those three things," he said. And becoming pregnant can lead to massive change in motivation for altering health behaviors in terms of diet, alcohol and drug intake, and smoking.

"It's because of a sudden change in identity," Gardner said. "They've suddenly become closely attuned to the risks of these behaviors." Reinforcing what has already been relayed, he said identity is one of the all-important mechanisms of behavior change; from it flows a set of rules. "If you see yourself as a particular person, then what does that person do?" he asked.

What does an expectant mother do?

I logged on to Facebook (Who am I kidding? I'm always logged on.) and made a single post asking for stories from women with addictions who then discovered they were pregnant. My inbox exploded.

"Lisa" wished to remain anonymous. At the age of twenty-two, she described herself as a heavy meth user who also drank several bottles of wine a day. She wrote that she "had been addicted to meth, alcohol, heroin, all sorts, since I was fifteen." She hasn't touched any drugs since learning she was pregnant eight years ago, although today she says she has the occasional glass of wine. She suffered physically from withdrawal when she quit, "but psychologically, the switch was very easy." She breastfed for two years as an added motivation to not slip back into old habits but said she never felt the pull again. In an instant upon learning there was a child growing inside her, she was done.

Victoria started drinking when she was eleven, then began smoking lots of pot. She became pregnant at sixteen, which, she said, "changed my life completely." She had been flunking out of school due to her addictions, but she instantly quit the booze and drugs when learning of her pregnancy. Now she has an eight-year-old daughter and is a year away from graduating from nursing school.

"Tracy" drank and smoked to excess and smoked marijuana frequently. She was also depressed. The night before she discovered she was pregnant, she was researching methods of suicide that were most effective. "The moment I got my positive test, I quit everything," she wrote. Feeling it wasn't just her life at stake, she said, "Ending my life wasn't an option anymore either." After her daughter was born, she took up running.

There were many other similar stories of women who had powerful addictions yet quit effortlessly because of a positive pregnancy test. Seeing that positive indicator on the pee-covered stick can flip a switch and change one's identity in an instant.

Identity governs how you behave, and the sudden thrust of motherhood upon a person can instantly make her proclaim, "I am not a smoker." Gardner refers to it as a simple and sudden psychological shift that makes withdrawal much easier to handle, because they have subscribed in full to the new identity.

In this regard, it's important to understand the difference between habit and behavior.

"To a psychologist, a habit is not something you do often," Gardner said. "It's something you do because it's become an automatic response to a particular situation." It's an adaptive process. And a person can still have a smoking habit but never smoke. "Someone may temporarily change their behavior, but they still have the habit with them." He explained how some women will begin smoking again after their child is born.

If someone's *habit* is to smoke first thing in the morning, that person requires a burst of motivation each morning to *not* do that, to consciously stop, each and every time. But when a pregnant woman wakes up in the morning, one of the first things that pops into her head is, *I'm pregnant.* This can stop the cigarette habit from entering her mind at all.

"That motivation, that ability, needs to be switched on at a critical point," Gardner said. The reason pregnancy is such a powerful tool is because it heightens that motivation and continuously makes them think about things differently.

He explained that psychological research isn't about breaking bad habits but more about stopping that habit from translating into behavior. The goal is to make the habit dormant. We are, all of us, walking around with dormant habits.

And a way to stop a habit from manifesting as behavior is to break the underlying association that triggers the action. Identity change has the power to break underlying associations. Gardner also expressed the value of doing something else to further break the association. "Being pregnant" is doing something, and so is being a mother.

If you didn't care about that little nugget of flesh growing inside you or creating an endless stream of poop once outside of you, such a thing wouldn't have much ability to alter identity and the rules such an identity creates for living. Yet we usually do care about our children. We love them, and that love transforms us.

Now if only they would clean their rooms.

"Walking with Peety"

Gilda Radner said, "I think dogs are the most amazing creatures; they give unconditional love. For me, they are the role model for being alive."

That "weird" friend who loves dogs more than people isn't so weird. A 2017 study of 256 people by researchers at Northeastern University in Boston found people were more empathetic toward stories of canine suffering than of that endured by humans. A partial explanation for why we're so enamored with the fuzzy quadrupeds has to do with their facial expressions. A 2017 study by researchers at the University of Portsmouth in England learned that dogs use a variety of expressions to communicate with humans. Even if said human is *not* holding a treat, they're trying to tell you something, and it brings us closer. One thing they might be trying to tell you is that they love you. A 2016 study published in *Social Cognitive and Affective Neuroscience* used fMRI technology on dogs and determined many value human praise even more than they value food. (Companionship dog breeds are more likely to value praise, whereas more independent "working" dogs place higher value on food.) And if you have siblings, you likely were accidentally called your brother's or sister's name by your parents many times. Interestingly, a 2016 study published in *Memory & Cognition* analyzed such "misnaming," finding that parents sometimes call their children by the dog's name too (but not the cat's), because we consider them to be part of the family.

I miss my dog.

And Eric O'Grey misses Peety, the dog who saved his life.

It's an inspiring tale that prompted a video created by the Humane Society of Silicon Valley. The video opens with Eric's voice: "In 2010, my doctor told me to buy a funeral plot, because I would need one within the next five years. But I'm still here, because a shelter dog saved my life."

Over one hundred million people have seen the video. *The New York Times* gave it top spot for "The Stories That Moved Us in 2016." If you decide to google "Eric and Peety," get the tissues ready.

Eric O'Grey's weight gain was "a slow and insidious process." He put on 150 pounds between the ages of twenty-five and fifty. His total cholesterol was over 400, what he referred to as "a walking dead level." His blood pressure was through the roof; it was painful to walk. His back and knees always ached. He tried to move as little as possible, getting food delivered to him through the window of his car or the door of his house.

Eric was unhealthy, depressed, and lonely. He had become a shut-in who had not been on a date in fifteen years. In 2010, he hit rock bottom while on a business flight.

The seat belt wouldn't fit over his frame, and the airline had run out of extenders. "I could hear people commenting around me that they were going to miss their connection because I was too fat." It was a miserable experience in which he felt like he'd become a burden. "I never wanted to do that," he said. "I had been a proud person."

Self-compassion remains important, but different people have different experiences, and Eric felt ashamed. This realization was his first holy-shit moment, but the biggest was yet to come.

He had tried several dozen weight-loss and fad diets. "Everything commercially marketed about weight loss, I had tried and failed on." Feeling somewhat primed for change from hitting bottom, the next day he recalled seeing President Bill Clinton being interviewed by Wolf Blitzer. Clinton looked leaner and more vibrant than he had in years and was extolling the virtues of a plant-based diet. O'Grey was on fifteen different medications for his various conditions: high cholesterol, high blood pressure, type 2 diabetes, depression. . . . He felt as though his physician wasn't offering him solutions to resolve the core issues, and was only treating symptoms. And so he googled to find an expert in plant-based eating nearby and set up an appointment with a nutrition expert.

The woman Eric met sat down with him for ninety minutes, listening to the problems of his life spill forth. She explained to him that you can mop the floor of an overflowing sink again and again, but you won't resolve the issue until you turn off the tap. O'Grey's primary issue, she said, was he'd become a recluse who had no friends and no joy in living. She gave him a simple, whole-food, plant-based diet and a prescription for a dog from the local shelter.

"I thought it was crazy to prescribe a dog." But she told him it would force him to go outside twice a day, get some sunshine, become more socialized. "I didn't believe it was going to work."

He went to a shelter in Silicon Valley, and the staff member in charge of adoptions spoke to him for an hour about why he wanted a dog. She reaffirmed a dog was a lifetime commitment; this was not a tryout. Eric told his tale, and she finally said, "I think I have the perfect dog for you."

Eric had visions of what would be a good dog for him. Something small and happy that was easy to take care of. "With all these visions dancing in my head, she walked in with this really large and unhealthy-looking dog." Peety had skin problems and was very overweight. He was an older dog who had trouble walking and looked unhappy.

"His head was hung low, looking at the ground, and when he looked up at me, it was the clearest sense of disappointment I'd ever seen on any creature in my life."

Eric was expecting something different, but so was Peety.

He was disappointed in his new dog, but the staff member had put a lot of thought into it, so he decided to trust her. She told Eric, "You're both in the same physical shape, and you need to partner to make both your lives healthier and happier."

He took Peety home, and for three days, they avoided each other. "This was a time of great reluctance," Eric told me. "I didn't really want to look after this dog."

For three days, they sat on opposite sides of the room from each other. For three days, they eyed each other skeptically. For three days, there was no life-changing moment for Eric O'Grey.

It was up to the dog to make the first move.

On the third night, Eric lay in bed. Living in a condo in San Jose, he had placed Peety's dog bed on the other side of his home from the bedroom. Eric awoke when he heard dog footsteps padding down the hall.

Peety leapt onto the bed. Eric was surprised such an out-of-shape dog could jump so high.

"That was the turning point," he said. At fifty years old, Eric had never had a pet. He'd never experienced bonding with an animal. The dog lay down next to him, and they looked into each other's eyes. "There was this deep, unconditional love that was more powerful than anything I'd ever felt before," he said. "We became best friends and truly bonded creatures in that moment. It changed everything for me."

Suddenly, he knew it was going to work. They were now accountability partners, dedicated to saving each other.

During the first few walks, they could only make it about a hundred yards before getting tired. After a couple of months, they were walking a few miles each time. "He loved me so much; he looked at me like I was the greatest person who ever walked the earth, so I decided to consciously become the person he thought I was." Eric followed the dietary advice he had been given and walked Peety every day.

Eric lost 150 pounds in ten months, eventually getting off all fifteen medications. Peety lost 25 pounds and became a vibrant and healthy dog. And he never returned to the dog bed; Peety slept in the same bed as Eric every night for the rest of his life.

The bonding between man and dog brought Eric out of his shell. The pair became known around the neighborhood and made friends during their walks. Feeling extra energy, Eric decided to join a local running group and made even more friends. "I started wondering if I could run a full marathon, and I felt like Peety was saying to me, 'Yeah, you can do this!' The dog had so much faith in me, I felt like I should have faith in myself." O'Grey ran as many as a hundred miles per week and qualified for the Boston Marathon.

But Peety grew older and developed cancer. Eric held his beloved dog in his arms as he passed. He still feels the loss.

Six months after Peety died, Eric was living in Washington State and, on a whim, stopped by the Seattle Humane Society. "I found Jake and we instantly bonded." Peety had loved his walks but hadn't enjoyed running.

Jake, however, knew how to run with his new human. Before long, the pair were doing trail runs up to eighteen miles.

But Eric still remembers that bond he first developed with Peety and how it changed his life. In 2017, O'Grey published a book, titled *Walking with Peety,* that details their story. Beyond the health changes, Eric advanced in his sales career, making more money than ever due to increased confidence, energy, and drive. He's happier than he's ever been, and the man who hadn't been on a date in fifteen years recently married.

I expect "Must love dogs" was part of Eric's requirement in finding a significant other.

Don't Hold Back Your Love

I got stuck at the end of the last section. I wasn't sure how to end this chapter. So, taking my own advice for achieving insight that is offered throughout this book, I engaged in diversion. I went outside for a run, and Hall & Oates came up on my iPod Shuffle.

"Don't Hold Back Your Love" is on my running playlist. Now you're judging me.

During the song, this entire conclusion was written in my head. Including that part. And this part. I'll stop now. (That part, too.)

Considering the growing gap in the world between "us" and "them," it's a tall order to follow Carl Rogers's advice of unconditional positive regard. Especially when "them" keeps acting like such dicks. Shit. Five minutes on Twitter and I'm thinking a rogue asteroid is exactly what this planet needs.

But perhaps there are people on your team. Perhaps you have an "us" you can derive inspiration from. Teams can motivate each other to greatness. There is also desire to be a good role model; those we love can instill a strong sense of duty we adhere to.

I didn't give you a task in the pregnancy section. "Oh, you want to break addiction and change your life? Go have a baby!" isn't advice I should be giving. I presented it as another indication of the identity-values model of self-control. When the title of "Mom" or "Dad" is thrust upon a person, amazing change can result.

Perhaps you need to get out there a bit more. It's what we're meant to do. Civilization wasn't built from hiding in caves. We are social creatures; we inspire each other to greatness.

Eric O'Grey had no one. Not a single friend. Then he found Peety. His situation didn't become "Me and you against the world," but "Me and you, *exploring* the world." They both made friends; they both had their lives changed through their loving partnership.

If you don't have a human to bond with right now, maybe a dog is the answer. I don't mean to piss off the cat people, but it's like Gilda said about that unconditional-love thing. If you seek it, a dog will provide. They are the epitome of viewing their humans with unconditional positive regard, which might explain why researchers at Manhattan College discovered via a 2016 study that dog ownership is associated with psychological benefits in terms of life satisfaction and "well-being."

It's a crime they leave us so soon, tickled to death by their own hearts.

Know that a dog is not a Bowflex; you can't shove one in the corner and use it for a coat rack. You must be a good human. Don't take this lifelong commitment lightly. If such a commitment seems too much, try volunteering to walk dogs at a local shelter as a start. You'll meet both four- and two-legged creatures. Who knows who you might fall in love with?

What do holy-shit moments do? They can do almost anything, but they're based on that core, *real* self, bursting to the surface. The part that has yearned to be recognized and set free. Such a moment comes with an overwhelming sense of rightness.

Rightness doesn't strike me as the type of thing built upon negative emotion. Open yourself; let love find a way.

You don't have to do this alone.

Act Now!

- Consider your love for the good people in your life, and endeavor to hold them in unconditional positive regard. In so doing, open yourself up to the breadth of human emotion rather than shutting down those feelings that may conflict with cognitive biases.

- Think of the future you have with those you love and how your hopes and dreams merge together. Ponder an ideal and seek to uncover what must happen today to bring that future to fruition.
- Reevaluate those relationships in need of it. If some are toxic and causing low self-worth, it may be time to consider alternatives. This will not be easy, but significant change never is.
- If you seek unconditional love, perhaps a dog is the answer, but do not take the commitment lightly. Be a good human.
- Open yourself to others. Let love find a way.

PART THREE

Hacking Epiphany

8

DREAMERS AREN'T DOERS: MAKING POSITIVE FANTASIES WORK FOR YOU INSTEAD OF AGAINST YOU

You don't have to be pushed. The vision pulls you.
—STEVE JOBS

It was the day before Canada Day 2011 in Vancouver, and I was happily going deaf.

I had entered an exclusive club: a few hours earlier I'd sat down with the media-shy drummer for Rush, Neil Peart, for a centerpiece feature in the *Los Angeles Times*. The band's representative gave me a pair of front row center tickets to the "Time Machine" tour that night.

"Time Machine" translates to "We're mostly playing the old stuff." Hell, yes.

I stand six feet tall. My best friend, Craig McArthur, is five feet ten. The thirteen-year-old boy Alex, immediately behind us, was about five feet four.

With his mother's permission, we brought him to the front row to stand between us. The kindly old security guard was making his rounds to check for wristbands on those in the front. When he saw Alex didn't have one I said, "We don't have a problem with him being up here." The man nodded. "If you don't have a problem, I don't have a problem." He walked on.

Alex loves Alex—Lifeson, that is, the band's guitar player. The boy turned his back to the stage and I snapped a photo of him with Lifeson in the background, then texted it to his mother.

I love Alex, too. And when I'm out for a run and hear the opening riff to "The Spirit of Radio," I imagine it's me playing.

I always wanted to be able to play guitar well. I tried to learn as a teen, but did not possess innate talent, and I also lacked the drive to overcome, via hard work, said absence of talent. I have a Fender acoustic sitting not far away, gathering dust. I could pick it up, search some videos on YouTube, and start learning again right now.

But it's a near certainty I won't. The fantasy of being an ace on guitar is more comforting than the years of effort it would take to master the instrument. Because I frequently daydream of having this amazing ability while my iPod or car stereo blares, I demotivate myself to log the hours to learn to do it. That's because dreamers aren't often doers.

Before I explain why: a confession. I hate the word "hacking."

Like with "quantum" and "self-actualization," it's been misused to promote things as epically stupid as heaping gobs of butter into overpriced coffee (barf), or even drinking your own urine (double barf). Much of what gets presented as hacking is bullshit. It's often a marketing term to sell crap.

Alas, I cannot think of a better descriptor for what I'm about to tell you.

Dammit.

Reevaluate Your Reality

We're trying to unlock a holy-shit moment to give you the sudden awakening and drive to pursue your dreams. The fact you're reading this book implies you are not, in fact, living the life of your dreams.

Doesn't mean it's all a shit sandwich.

Could suck. Could be a "good to great" situation. The key point is, life isn't where you want it to be, and you're seeking sudden change.

Why?

What's the problem? This is the first step in hacking epiphany. Ugh. You know what? I'm going to not use that word, like, *ever* again. As discussed previously, you must develop discrepancy and generate inner conflict—conflict between how things are and have been, and how you wish them to be. Seek that which is wrong. Examine it and endeavor to crystallize the various pieces of discontent that permeate your life. Crystallization of dis-content will vary from person to person. If you're good seeking great, it's about reaching a tipping point. If it's poop on pumpernickel, it's more about the *breaking* point.

I'm not trying to break you, but if aspects of the hitting-rock-bottom stuff sound uncomfortably familiar, you know you can't continue in the same vein. Change goes against our nature. We need a good reason to do it, so this task is about seeking those good reasons.

History is not destiny.

The myriad tragedies of life can render many unable to cope; there is no shame in this. And yet there may be untapped resilience lying within, ready to do battle with the past and secure a better future.

Boris Cyrulnik is a French psychiatrist whose Jewish parents were murdered by Nazis during the Second World War. He was born in 1937, and his childhood was one of immense suffering, both during and after the war. It led him to study how trauma and suffering can contribute to the *making* of someone rather than the undoing.

He showed that the human brain is malleable; it can recover if we allow it. A child can suffer trauma, and brain scans show this results in shrinking of the cerebral ventricles and cortex. But with the loving care of others, a traumatized person's brain can recover and return to normal. In his 2009 book *Resilience,* Cyrulnik writes, "Resilience is a mesh and not a substance. We are forced to knit ourselves, using the people and things we meet in our emotional and social environments." Resilience is not a character trait we're born with, where some have more, and others, less. It's something we create; it's a process requiring the right conditions.

One of those conditions is the care of others. The simple feeling of compassion from those who are close to you is a boon to those seeking inner strength to battle past suffering. There was good reason for writing the previous chapter.

You may feel overwhelmed, lost, punished by your past. You may benefit from a reevaluation of yourself and the world around you. Twentieth-century French philosopher Maurice Merleau-Ponty wrote in 1945 of our need to "break with our familiar acceptance" of the world. How we view our past is not often an accurate portrayal of how things were or are. Merleau-Ponty was a fan of questioning our assumptions of what was and what is, looking at the world with fresh eyes to see with clarity where we may go from here.

Imagine you are an outside observer of yourself, your life, and your situation. Without all your mental baggage in tow, what would you imagine could be possible of such a person if they were truly inspired?

That was a task. This chapter is full of them. Keep an eye out.

Raise Consciousness and Respond Accordingly

It need not be only you engaged in objective analysis.

"Consciousness-raising" is about increasing your awareness of personal issues. A place to start can be a visit to your family physician. If you have current or impending health problems, a medical professional can run tests and provide feedback based on quantitative data. This may involve taking a closer look at where you're spending time and effort and focusing more on self-care rather than always being a caretaker for others. If you're run down and your health is suffering, your ability to contribute to the benefit of those you care for will also suffer.

You may need to put yourself first. If you are a woman, and especially if you are a mother, odds are you're bad at this. Except it's not you who is bad, it's the societal construct. A 2002 study by researchers at the University of Michigan found "normative female gender role responsibilities such as childcare and housework" lead to lower levels of physical activity and less focus on making one's health a priority. These barriers persist even for women living with chronic illness, because they are still too focused on the care of others.

Self-care is not selfish. It's why the airline tells you to put your oxygen mask on first. If others have a high level of dependency on you, an intervention may be necessary. If you are to be able to continue helping them, they must in turn help you by allowing you freedom for self-care.

Another consideration is psychotherapy. If you're already in it, ascertain if you've lapsed into "therapeutic inertia." Ken Resnicow refers to this as "an insidious and powerful force in which both patients and their providers stop trying to innovate." Together, you have come to believe you're never getting better. And if this is the case, it's time to "change the initial conditions," Resnicow says, tying back to his fondness for chaos theory. That could mean finding a new therapist to look at you and your issues with fresh eyes. Or starting from scratch with your current provider.

Consciousness-raising is key in identity change. Again, you need to get emotional and consider how you feel about yourself. Do you feel like a "couch potato"? What are the benefits to changing that? Do a bit of delving into the research and look at what big-picture benefits could accrue from engaging in new activities. What happens when you exercise? What happens when you eat better? What happens when you quit smoking? What happens when you go back to school / change your career / spend more time with family / find a new hobby / find love? Imagine what's on the other side of the holy-shit moment.

It all takes effort, but as Jim Collins writes in *Good to Great,* it's about being "rigorous, not ruthless." This is striving to be your focused best, not killing yourself to achieve some impossible, externally proffered "ideal."

Raise your consciousness, become more mindful of your current situation, and perhaps have "a baby epiphany" to kick things off. That's what Ellen Langer calls the process of engaging in mindfulness. "You learn to stop acting in a robotic way," she said. Then she told me a story about a horse.

It was long ago, she was at a horse-racing event, and a trainer asked Langer to watch his horse so he could go buy a hotdog. For the horse. She spoke to me of her Yale and Harvard education and how it made her believe she knew it all. As I mentioned earlier, Langer was the first woman to become a tenured professor of psychology at Harvard. And, knowing horses are herbivores, she thought the man ridiculous. "He comes back, and the horse eats the hotdog," she said. "At that moment, I realized everything I 'knew' could be wrong."

Then she began to question. The questioning meant she didn't immediately accept limits other people saw as real. It made her realize many have an "illusion of certainty," which she considers mindlessness by another term.

"Whatever it is that wakes us up, once we are awake, we notice."

This is the essence of mindfulness, of paying attention and reevaluating. Of gathering information and raising your consciousness. It is a simple process of noticing new things, and in so doing, realizing you didn't know things as well as you thought you did.

It opens myriad possibilities.

That which was boring can become interesting again. Suddenly, you find opportunities where you were blind to them before. It's about being *responsive* to the world rather than *reactive*. When you feel reactive, you're not perceiving much choice for how to deal with a given situation: If it's something good, you feel compelled to have it. If it's something bad, you are driven to do away with it. You've removed your ability to choose how you respond by allowing your past to dictate your current behavior.

Responsiveness is about you being in charge rather than some external reality, Langer told me. "Nothing is fated. Control your own destiny."

Rather than react, stop. Investigate. Consider your options. Respond accordingly.

Dream Appropriately

When it comes to ever learning to play guitar, my dreaming sucks.

You can dream about a better future, but if you do it the wrong way, it's counterproductive to achieving it. In chapter 1, I mentioned the work of Professor Gabriele Oettingen on how we need to rethink positive thinking. Time for a closer look.

"Dreaming about the future makes people *less* likely to realize their dreams and wishes," she writes in *Rethinking Positive Thinking*. Fantasizing doesn't lead to achievement, rather it mires us in indecision and apathy.

But I thought we were just supposed to think happy thoughts, then the universe would throw cool shit at us. If that's the case, I guess the millions of people who die from starvation each year didn't think positively enough to "attract" food.

Oettingen first came to realize the problems associated with excessive fantasizing about the future in 1991, when she studied twenty-five women with obesity enrolled in a weight-loss program. She presented them with several future scenarios to ascertain how they felt about the program and their lives after completing it. A year later, the results were fascinating.

The women who believed they were likely to lose weight were far more successful than those who didn't think they would lose weight. So far, positive thinking appears a great thing. But there's more. Those who were successful did so because they were *dreaming appropriately* about how to achieve the goal, by focusing on overcoming barriers. The unsuccessful ones engaged in pure fantasy, dreaming about what it would be like to achieve the goal, creating images of a slimmer physique and how attractive they might feel. *Such achievement fantasies impeded doing the work to get the results.*

Oettingen faced backlash from the scientific community. How dare she question the power of positive thinking?

Nevertheless, she persisted. Working with colleague Doris Mayer out of the University of Hamburg, they published a compilation of four studies in 2002. In it, they evaluated graduates seeking employment, students with a crush on a fellow student, students anticipating an upcoming exam, and patients about to undergo hip-replacement surgery.

It was the same kind of study, to ascertain motivation to work toward a goal (getting a job, a date, a high grade, or successful post-surgical rehab) based on the participant's attitudes going into it. The results? Positive *expectations* = good. Positive *fantasies* = not good.

In other words, when you "expect" to work and you focus on what is needed to achieve and you have confidence in your abilities to do so, you're gonna kick some ass. Conversely, when you focus on daydreaming about how awesome life will be once said goal is achieved, it saps your willpower to do . . . anything.

Why?

Because in your mind, you already kind of achieved it.

In my mind, when I'm out for a run and imagining what an amazing guitar player I am, fingers twitching to that righteous solo, I'm immersed in an imaginary sense of achievement. It's relaxing, and therefore the *good stress* needed to *do the work* to achieve the goal in the first place is removed. Oettingen and Mayer explain that positive fantasies "lead people to mentally enjoy the desired future in the here and now."

Without having to work for it.

Good to Great has an extreme example of this, referred to as "The Stockdale Paradox." It's the tale of Admiral Jim Stockdale, the highest ranking American officer imprisoned in the "Hanoi Hilton" during the Vietnam War. Taken in 1965, he was tortured over twenty times during the next eight years. But he made it home.

Many of his fellow prisoners did not.

Author Jim Collins asked Admiral Stockdale about those who never got to come home. "The optimists," he replied. Collins was confused, because moments before, Stockdale had said he never lost faith that he would make it home. The admiral elaborated: the "optimists" were the ones who said they'd be home by Christmas, but then Christmas would come and go. Then they would say, "home by Easter," and that holiday would also pass, yet they remained imprisoned under horrible conditions.

Admiral Stockdale said such men died of broken hearts.

Then he offered this advice to Collins: "You must never confuse faith that you will prevail in the end—which you can never afford to lose—with the discipline to confront the most brutal facts of your current reality, whatever they might be."

Although it was two decades prior to Gabriele Oettingen beginning her research in this area, what allowed Stockdale to persevere is in line with her findings.

My personal transformation is so lightweight in comparison to the trials of Admiral Stockdale it is barely worth mentioning, but it's my book. Years ago, I faced the reality I was lazy, and the mess I was in was of my own making. Part of my realization was that I worked hard at being lazy. There were tasks each day that I had to engage in mental gymnastics to shirk. Rather than receive a dopamine boost from progress, I felt each failure of effort at a personal level. I was unable to enjoy my laziness. With my sudden epiphany about needing to work, there was the reality I was already putting effort into indolence, and a profound redirection of energy was required.

The barrier to my success contained the answer to overcoming it.

"Focus on the journey, not the destination" is such a cliché, but sometimes clichés come about for good reason. That being written, positive fantasies are not all bad, especially if they're the result of high expectations of success. When you're doing the work and feeling invigorated about how well it's going, it's okay to dream a little about how awesome that goal achievement will be.

So, what to do?

After an additional decade of research, Oettingen published another study examining how positive fantasies can *wisely* be used for goal attainment. And, yes, this relates to epiphany. We're getting to it.

It starts with a wish.

"Come up with a wish that is dear to you," Professor Oettingen told me. When we go through everyday life, she explained, we don't often think of the wishes that have deep meaning for us, because we just respond to the environment. Ellen Langer cautions against that reactionary, mindless living. The goal is to come up with *your* wish, a real wish that is not what you believe other people think you should be striving for, but what your deepest desires hold true for you.

A wish that is based upon the true self, it must flow out of your core identity and values.

How to find it? "Allow yourself a bit of calm and focus," Oettingen said in a soothing voice. She says to relax, take some time, and just . . . think. Keep your wish to three or four words about what you would most desire. Think about your most positive possible outcome. "Keep it in front of your mind and allow yourself to imagine and experience the outcome," she said. "Just let your mind go and ponder that."

Easier said than done? If you can't imagine this at your current stage, we'll take it to the next level in the next chapter. Either way, it's only part of the process of wielding a machete to carve a path through the epiphany jungle. (I told you I wasn't using that "h" word any longer.)

Seek the Obstacle

The impediment to action advances action.
What stands in the way becomes the way.
—DUMBLEDORE?

My mother was in love with Richard Harris. Even though he sang that horrible "MacArthur Park" song. Her desire for him arose from the 1970 film *A Man Called Horse.* I thought he made the better Dumbledore. Alas, he moved on into the great unknown after only two *Harry Potter* films.

Joaquin Phoenix killed him.

In *Gladiator,* I mean; that multiple-Oscar-winning movie about second-century Italians with English accents. Harris played Emperor Marcus Aurelius. It was Aurelius who said that stuff about the impediment to action and what stands in the way, so you could say Dumbledore . . . Never mind.

Aurelius was a real emperor, and he did kick quite a bit of northern European ass. He often wrote on stoic philosophy, and this was compiled into a book titled *Meditations* after his death. That's where the quote comes from, in the fifth book—although the modernized quote has been made punchier than the translation I read, cutting words like "doth" and "readiest."

This is another example of Oettingen's research reflecting history. In her 2012 study published in the *European Review of Social Psychology,* she analyzed the way we view the future and how this affects behavior change. In it, Oettingen discussed a "metacognitive strategy" for contrasting visions of the desired future with the *resisting* reality to produce active goal pursuit. She calls it "mental contrasting." It starts with finding the right goal and understanding its outcome, the "wish" discussed in the previous section. Next, Oettingen says, you must determine what is stopping you from achieving the wish. This is the setup for epiphany to strike. You did the part of finding what you want, fantasized a little about how wonderful achievement will be, but now it's time "to circumvent the calming effects of dreaming and mobilize dreams as a tool for prompting directed action." Copy that? *Mobilize* those dreams!

"Find the main obstacle that stands in your way," Oettingen told me.

"You'll have to dig deep." She explained this with the example of "lack of time" for pursuing a specific goal, which then requires uncovering *why* you don't have time and what could be reprioritized to provide it. It may be lack of organization, or anxiety over capabilities, or whether you feel as though you deserve to do something for you. . . .

Recall the expectancy-value approach, discussed in chapter 1: choosing an ambitious goal (has high value), but one that is achievable (you *expect* to be able to do it if you work hard enough). Part of what mental contrasting does, after finding a goal of high value, is to reveal the obstacle and determine how to work through it. Once you find your "What stands in the way becomes the way," you're energized because expectancy explodes. You now comprehend the *wise* pursuit of this goal.

But what if the way is revealed as impossible?

Oettingen writes in her 2012 paper that uncovering *impossibility* comes with its own benefits. "It de-energises people when their wishes are beyond their reach, thus promoting disengagement, freeing people for alternative pursuits."

If it's impossible, it wasn't the right goal. Not the droids you're looking for. Move along. Oettingen told me this freeing allows people to let go of a goal with a clear conscience. Because of the realization of the lack of achievability, failure to attain no longer plagues. It means you have increased clarity to focus on a more appropriate and attainable goal.

What if the goal is not impossible, but merely implausible? This can give you a giant kick in the ass. Remember, I'm a fan of chasing the implausible. *Lofty* goals are awesome, so long as you ground them in reality. Dolly Parton said, "You need to really believe in what you've got to offer, what your talent is—and if you believe, that gives you strength." Who are you to deny Dolly?

"When they find that main obstacle that is holding them back, people often have an epiphany," Oettingen told me. "They finally realize, *Yes! This is it! This is what has been preventing me from fulfilling my wish.*"

She explained that this is an opening of a path, where suddenly, people know what to do, where to go. The positive fantasy provides initial direction; finding the obstacle and how to overcome it—to turn it into *the way*—is what energizes, so they feel compelled. *When you learn how to conquer that obstacle, you come to feel as though you must.*

Professor Oettingen said this "is not a rational process whatsoever." Finding the wish is emotional. It's an imagination exercise intended to generate passionate pursuit. "Once you find the obstacle and how to overcome it, this can be a very emotional experience because you finally know what's been hampering you." Sometimes this obstacle has been in your way for years, yet you never realized it. Sometimes it's not a flattering thing you learn about yourself, what this obstacle was. But it *is* unburdening.

Activate Appetite

Be open to new experiences.

In 2003, researchers from the University of Rochester examined "inspiration as a psychological construct." They described openness to experience using an interesting word I'd not read before: "appetitive." Hmmm. I was expecting spell-check to flag that. Go Microsoft.

Anyway, appetitive. Being *hungry* for new experience. And sudden, life-changing epiphany is one helluva new experience. You must *want* this and believe it can come to you. Professor Resnicow warns to watch out for counter-arguing, which can happen when you're trying too hard to persuade yourself. It's important to let the appetite for new experience flow through you like the Force, young Jedi, rather than trying to strong-arm it. If it doesn't feel right, you'll fight back.

As Ellen Langer explains in *Mindfulness,* it's important not to mindlessly believe in the limits we place upon ourselves. The more mindful of your talents you become, the more open to future possibility you are.

Set the stage, open yourself, hungrily; perhaps look at the sky.

Still think epiphany can't be (that word I won't use)? In *The Eureka Factor,* Kounios and Beeman tell the story of Greg Swartz, director of innovation for Ping, a maker of golf equipment, on how he primes his mind for sudden enlightenment.

Swartz stressed the importance of doing one's homework beforehand.

You need to spend a lot of time working the problem via analysis prior to setting up the lightning rod and waiting for something to strike it. When he's of a mind to seek insight to resolve a problem, Swartz waits until night, but not too late; relaxed, yet not ready for sleep. He gathers some minimal information about the problem—which in his case was how to improve golf-club design—then goes outside, plays some nondistracting background music, lies back in a comfortable chair, and looks at the night sky, gazing past the stars and on into infinity.

He then ponders what he's looking for in the most general sense, yet without thinking in a deliberate or methodical manner. He allows thoughts to "meander and collide."

When the right idea strikes, he suddenly changes tack, from unfocused to focused, analyzing the idea and formulating how to enact it. This "planning," by the way, is the final step in Oettingen's approach. Once the way past the obstacle is ascertained and you are energized, this is when you begin to work out the details using System 2.

MAKE IT HAPPEN!

You're going to need to set some time aside to do this. Rather than taking a break now, I recommend opening your electronic calendar to set a specific time to follow through on Professor Oettingen's instructions. Mood state is important; choose a time and location you can relax in. Reread the above section regarding how Greg Swartz sets the stage for creative enlightenment, and consider replicating circumstances you believe are helpful.

When you are all ready, work to find your true wish. *Your* wish, not what others expect. When that is accomplished, consider the most positive outcome. Keep it in the front of your mind and allow yourself to experience it. Now seek the obstacle, that which is stopping you from achieving this wish. Dig deep and seek the reasons *why* this obstacle exists. Find the way through that obstacle, or, if the wish is deemed impossible, discard it with a clear conscience and move on to something else.

Work your way through the problem of bursting through that barricade. Entice the lightning to strike and help you solve the problem. When inspiration arrives, switch to System 2 and get busy planning. It may not happen the first few times you try it. But with practice, you can get better, find your way forward, and become energized.

Comprehending Capabilities

Can you be Dumbledore? Or Marcus Aurelius. Or whomever?

In the introduction I wrote of past performance accomplishments, a parameter of self-efficacy theory. I asked if you'd had a previous epiphany. Now we must examine your capabilities for overcoming obstacles.

So, think on that.

Achieving implausible dreams requires tenacity. When have you shown it before? When was there a mighty roadblock and you blasted through it, either with a massive surge or a slow-and-steady yet deliberate movement forward?

Because if you've done it before, you can do it again. And the more similar the past experience to the future goal, the better. Ponder that. Be energized by the confidence it imbues.

If you lack such experience, others have it.

Vicarious experiences present another parameter of self-efficacy, also referred to as "modeling." Find someone who has done what you desire to do, and take education and inspiration from them. The more this person is similar to you, the better. It's also advantageous if you know this person, but it's not required. It can be a celebrity or public figure, if you wish.

Assess your pain tolerance. Imagine it's Sean Connery in *The Untouchables,* asking, "What are you prepared to do?"

The way will not be easy. Yet you embrace the challenge because it has become your passion, where work comes to feel like play. I'll amend Connery's line: What are you prepared to *become passionate about*?

Frame the Way Forward

In *Thinking, Fast and Slow,* Daniel Kahneman writes of framing effects. An example he gives is that odds of surviving a surgery being 90 percent sounds *way better* than saying the surgery presents a 10 percent chance of death.

Consider the odds of success, not failure.

But remember to use System 2 not just for confirmation but for finding the footsteps. System 1 creates the epiphany, and System 2 shows the way. It's the analytical system that helps create the plan, but recall it also needs to be kept in check. I mentioned a 2011 study examining "feelings as information," which found that overanalyzing the rightness of the decision can make things less appealing because it kills the emotional force driving you forward. It's important here to repeat the KISS acronym: *Keep it simple, stupid.* This is especially true when it comes to the benefits of change. Focus on the big picture and work through the details as needed.

Another method Kahneman recommends is to consider the outside view. This is again about being objective regarding your capabilities and your way forward. Imagine what an outsider would tell you to do. Also, imagine *you* are the outsider looking at a person in your situation. Examine this imaginary twin and ask what advice you would give him or her.

In all of this, hold on to optimism. It is what will see you through when things get tough.

Because they will get tough.

Script with Simplicity

In *Switch,* the Heath brothers write, "What looks like resistance is often a lack of clarity." The example they use, eating a healthier diet, is challenging when you don't know what "healthier diet" means. And yet, as I pointed out in the previous section, too much information is as bad as not enough. Keep it simple, but not too minimal, and not obscure.

Chip and Dan Heath want you to "script the critical moves."

"Ambiguity is the enemy," they state. It's exhausting to have to evaluate multiple options. Ensure your road ahead is clear. If it's unclear, you'll default to your usual behaviors. Find the critical moves that motivate you to achieve your goal—the most simple and clear way to transform what stands in the way, *into* the way.

Another bit of advice from the Heath brothers is "Shrink the change."

This directly relates to the role of dopamine in providing ongoing motivation to persevere. Dopamine recognizes progress, and even minimal progress gives a hit of that rewarding neuromodulator you crave. Shrinking the change is a way to evaluate your continual progress. It's more of that cliché journey-not-destination stuff. You may still be many miles from your goal, but dopamine cares about the steps you took today.

Don't forget to stop, look at, and examine those steps. Take pride in them. Feel the neurochemical positive-reinforcement flow.

Act Now!

- Imagine you are an outside observer of your life. Ditch the mental baggage for a moment and endeavor to be fully objective. Imagine what would be possible for this person—you—if you became *inspired*.

- If health issues are a potential concern, begin consciousness-raising with a visit to your physician. Seek feedback from a medical professional based on quantitative data about the current state of your health for consideration in the way forward.

- Self-care is not selfish. If an intervention is needed to reduce dependency on you so you can look after yourself, do it.

- Beware therapeutic inertia. Evaluate if you and your provider have stopped innovating and come to believe you're never getting better. If this is the case, consider switching to a new provider or starting from scratch with your current one to re-examine things with fresh eyes.

- Gather information about the benefits of change in the areas you are interested in: health, addiction, education, employment, relationships, etc.

- Practice mindfulness by pausing to think. Rather than always being reactive, don't consider you are fated to do anything. Imagine the myriad possibilities and be *responsive* in the way that seems most appropriate. Control your own destiny.
- Come up with a wish that is dear to *you,* not one other people believe you should be striving for. Take some time and relax to let it flow as a general, big picture of what you'd like to accomplish.
- Take that wish and spend a little time having a positive fantasy about the outcome. Consider the many benefits of what life will be like once you've achieved it.
- Recall your past performance accomplishments for which you pushed through roadblocks. Understand that because you have done it before, you can do it again.
- Engage in vicarious experience by finding a model who has done what you are trying to do. Gain inspiration and even take guidance from that person.
- Mobilize your dreams by working to find the main obstacle that stands in the way of achieving them. You'll have to dig deep, so consider setting aside a specific time when you can relax without distraction to let ideas "meander and collide" to achieve sudden insight. This is where epiphany can strike. Be ready for it. Remember, you need to do your homework beforehand. You need to be primed for enlightenment by first having spent time on analysis.
- Watch out for counterarguing. Let the appetite for new experience flow through you rather than trying to force it. If you try too hard to persuade yourself—if it doesn't feel right— you'll fight back.
- If your dream is revealed as impossible, move on with a clear conscience to something else.
- Frame the way forward in a positive light by considering the likelihood of success rather than dwelling on odds of failure.

- If the solution to overcoming your primary obstacle arrives, switch from insight to analysis. Engage System 2 to work out the details, but remember to keep it simple by focusing on the most important details. Avoid ambiguity and "script the critical moves."
- "Shrink the change" by focusing on progress. Take pride in small wins, and get that dopamine hit.

Postscript to Chapter 8

I have said this is not necessarily a weight-loss book, but perhaps that is your dream. Consider the possibility that, while you are using these methods, the dream is revealed as impossible.

That can happen.

I wrote an article titled "'Eat Less, Move More' Is Bullshit," and it was named the number-one fat-loss article of the year for 2016 by the Personal Trainer Development Center. It was *not* a denial of calories in vs. calories out. I would never say that anything other than a caloric deficit leads to weight loss. *But!* There is so much involved in a person's life that has significant impact on how many calories that person burns and consumes. The solution to obesity can't be boiled down to a sound bite. Doing so is a form of fat shaming; it makes it seem so simple anyone can do it, when it's anything but.

People like Chuck Gross and Eric O'Grey succeeded with significant weight loss after multiple failed attempts, but that doesn't mean it's possible for everyone. Obesity is a multifactorial condition, and "eat less, move more" is the grossest oversimplification of how to solve the problem, to the point of being ridiculous. Genetics, injuries, illnesses, medication, past trauma, life situation, financial struggles—there are so many factors that can make sustained weight loss such a challenge, that for some it can appear impossible.

And yet, people continue to try, repeatedly, even when the effort is making them miserable.

There are those in the body-acceptance movement who deny the health risks associated with obesity. They're wrong. I am a big fan of body accep-tance, but it is an unfortunate reality that excess body fat is often associ-ated with negative impact on health.

But consider the impact on your psyche of constantly trying and failing to lose weight.

Do you not deserve happiness? Do you not deserve to *flourish*?

If you seek that obstacle to weight loss for all you're worth, and if your situation is such that you determine it is impossible, that's the way it is. Stop letting repeated failure at weight loss make you miserable. Love your body for what it can do, take care of it the best you can, and go out there and kick ass at something else. Perhaps it will become possible one day in the future. Don't let it put your life on hold now.

There is so much more to life than numbers on a scale.

9

NUDGING TOWARD THE LEAP:
BATTLING THE STATUS QUO AND PREPARING YOUR
MIND FOR EPIPHANY

The most common way people give up their power
is by thinking they don't have any.
—ALICE WALKER

have asked whichever child moves out of the house last to present me
with a sock. That way, I can run around the house, waving the sock,
crying, "Dobby is a free elf!"

Hopefully they'll stay moved out. My wife and I are planning to launch
these two far enough they'll not find their way home. Not throwing them
to the wolves, per se, but ensuring they have the tools to succeed. We've
spent years preparing them.

There is much to be said for careful preparation. As mentioned earlier,
"Inspiration favors the prepared mind."

Just because epiphany is something that pops in doesn't mean you can't
plan for it, both mentally and practically, preparing yourself for life-changing
insight to arrive. You may not be able to determine "when" it will happen,
but there is plenty of strategic work to be done to skew the odds regarding
"if" it will.

I know a doctor who was ready for it.

He is an in-demand specialist, often running from patient to patient.
In 2009, as we were finishing up, he said, "How is everything else going?"

"It's good," I said. "I'm transitioning my career toward being a full-time health-and-fitness writer."

"Really?" he said, intrigued, then grabbed his prodigious belly. "Inspire me!"

I thought for moment. We'd left his office and were standing in the hallway. I knew I had about thirty seconds—the time allotted for what they call in the business world the "elevator pitch," where you need to give someone the gist, quickly, to sell them on a concept; it must hit the supreme highlights and get them excited.

I was new at this but had an inkling. This was my pitch:

"Do some homework and seek to find an activity you can become passionate about. Throw time and effort and even money into it. Just keep trying to get better. Even let it come to define you as a person so this new activity becomes a part of who you are." I stopped, thinking what I'd said was pretty good, then realized I'd forgotten the most important part, since he was interested in weight loss. "Don't forget to fuel appropriately."

He appeared pensive, then said, "That's good stuff."

I didn't see him for a year.

In 2010, I sat in his office again; he was transformed. At least forty pounds lighter, much fitter, more energized. I suspected he wanted to tell me about his transformation but was holding back because I was the patient. It was my time.

At the end of the appointment, I stood and turned toward the door. Hanging on the wall, I saw a framed photo. It was of the doctor, decked out in body armor and riding a fancy mountain bike down a steep grade.

I nodded toward the photo. "Nice bike."

"Thanks!" he replied with enthusiasm. Then, more somber: "Seriously. Thank you."

It worked, in part, because he was ready to take my advice. He was waiting for sudden inspiration.

So was Sarah.

I published the story of the mountain-biking doctor on my website in January 2017. The following November, I posted the link on Facebook again, because traffic = advertising revenue. Sarah wrote in the comments on the second posting that reading the article earlier in the year had prompted her to register for a "couch to 5K" running program. Ten months later, she was getting ready to run her first half marathon, with no intention of stopping.

These people were nudged toward sudden change. It worked because they were *ready* to be nudged. The previous chapters have been about getting you ready, the planning and preparation. If epiphany hasn't happened yet, let's see what we can do about making the final push.

Avoiding "Yeah, Whatever"

In chapter 3, I quoted Cass Sunstein and referred to his work on what Daniel Kahneman refers to as the "bible of behavioral economics." The book *Nudge* was coauthored with University of Chicago professor Richard Thaler, who won the Nobel Memorial Prize in Economic Sciences in 2017.

Nudge examines strategies that governments and organizations can enact to get you to do stuff that's both good for you and for others while maximizing freedom of choice. That second part makes it seem less *1984*-ish, I guess.

When I was young and refueling my 1981 Honda Accord, I left the gas cap on top of the car and drove away. It cost thirty-five dollars to replace, which in 1985 dollars was a lot of money to teenage James. There was much profanity.

I'd made a "postcompletion error." One example of a "nudge" is the inclusion of a few cents' worth of plastic to attach the gas cap to the vehicle so this doesn't happen. The routine used to be placing the gas cap on top of the car, which invited mistakes of leaving it behind. With this simple change, the routine changes and the errors are avoided. Another such nudge some companies implemented to improve "consumer welfare" was to make the diesel nozzle too big to fit inside the fuel receptacle of gasoline engines. You want to talk expensive mistakes? Try driving a Mustang using diesel. This is part of what Thaler and Sunstein refer to as "choice architecture." That piece of plastic changed the default routine, preventing us from leaving the expensive gas cap behind, and the bigger nozzle made it impossible to incorrectly fuel a vehicle.

Changing defaults is an important part of choice architecture. Otherwise, we are likely to engage in what the authors refer to as the "yeah, whatever" heuristic. A heuristic is a practical way of doing things that is not necessarily optimal, but a strategy derived from previous ways of getting the job done, more or less.

I used to do this making teriyaki chicken wings: for years, I would place the wings onto a baking sheet, then pour the thick glaze from the wide-mouth bottle onto each individual wing, then brush it around with a basting brush. It was time-consuming, messy, and wasteful, but it got the job done. One day, it suddenly occurred to me I could pour the glaze into a bowl, dip the brush into the bowl, and spread it onto the wings. (Before you say toss the wings in the bowl, understand the glaze is too thick for that.)

I never said I was a great cook. Most of what I know is by trial and error.

Anyway, the latter is a far superior method. It's faster, uses less, makes less mess. Had it never occurred to me, my default of the less effective, messier way would continue to be used. Because yeah, whatever.

Thaler and Sunstein refer to these defaults as "ubiquitous and powerful," and unless we adopt strategies to break the routine, we'll continue the same less optimal methods and approaches to doing things, and to living.

It goes beyond basting chicken wings and into what is called the "status quo bias." First uncovered in 1988 by researchers at Boston and Harvard Universities, it's the tendency to stick with the status quo in decision-making, even when being presented with a better option involving change. What's more, we tend to rationalize not changing, because you're not the boss of me. Either that, or we do nothing and let the status quo prevail. Part of this also has to do with loss aversion being much more motivating than potential gain.

Thaler and Sunstein gave an example of how status quo bias is exploited with the free magazine subscription that begins charging your credit card after three months. Free sounds great, even though you never read the magazine and then neglect to cancel the subscription even after years of being charged for it and not reading it.

Yeah, whatever.

Fear of change *is* ubiquitous, and it is powerful. Eighteenth-century English essayist Samuel Johnson said, "To do nothing is in every man's power." An ingrained human desire to maintain the status quo, to avoid loss, can keep you mired in a mediocre life. We cannot rely on others to nudge us toward a sudden, inspired leap of dramatic change.

We must learn to nudge ourselves.

No Safe Battles

That's another Churchill quote: "Success cannot be guaranteed. There are no safe battles."

Get over it. Or tiptoe safely to death. Your call.

If you seek to expose the greatness lying within, fear of failure must be conquered, or at least ameliorated. One way to do so is oft-repeated in these pages: *analyze*! Do the pre-work. Get the confirmation from System 2 and put it to work on how to best implement change. Competence creates confidence.

Despite there being much risk and no guarantee of success, I knew I wanted to leave the corporate world and become a writer. I also knew my income would take a hit, likely for years (I was right about that). What's more, I knew if I tried for years, and failed, it would be next to impossible to get back on the previous career track. Fear of loss was palpable. But once the inspiration for massive career change struck, there was no denying the quest. When the opportunity arose to make the leap, I told my wife, "If I don't try this, I'm going to die."

She has always been my biggest supporter. But I didn't leap without a plan. And the plan kept changing, kept adapting based on new information, and eventually . . . *success*!

I was ready to take those risks, make that leap, not just from being inspired, but because I'd used System 2 to analyze. This made the inspiration *convincing*. It wasn't a whim, but a calculated risk worth taking. I also knew I was ready to work my ass off to bring it to fruition, I was that passionate.

I was passionate because I was informed about the path ahead; my perceived odds of success and potential payoff overshadowed fear of loss.

Rosa Parks said, "Knowing what must be done does away with fear." Add to this, Dale Carnegie: "Inaction breeds doubt and fear. Action breeds confidence and courage." Seek the knowledge *and* passion that prompt action, growing your confidence.

And your courage.

Break Your Programming

"Man is defined as a human being and woman as a female."

These are the words of existentialist philosopher and feminist Simone de Beauvoir, published in her 1949 book, *The Second Sex,* in response to Sigmund Freud's view of women as inferior beings. The quote continues on to explain that when a woman behaves as a human, she is said to be imitating men.

Freud, like Churchill, was a man of his time: bigoted as all hell. Such sexism still permeates society. The previous chapter exposed how some women fail at self-care because "normative female gender role responsibilities" practically force them to put others first. And yet, certain "men's rights" groups proclaim feminism took gender equality and "swung the pendulum too far the other way."

I hate those guys. I wrote about them for *TIME* magazine; the piece blew up and got a positive mention on CNN TV. You should see the hate mail.

Regardless of gender and inherent societal constructs and programming, there is room for choice. Alas, an authentic existence true to one's self means breaking with the status quo you are biased toward upholding. There is risk associated with denying the role society foists upon you.

There is also freedom.

When you seek such freedom from what the world says you *must* do, what it *expects* you to do and be, and instead open yourself to possibilities lying outside what is considered normal or appropriate, your potential vision for the future is made boundless.

Malala Yousafzai, a young Pakistani activist for women's rights, said, "We cannot all succeed when half of us are held back." *Don't hold back*. Add to this the advice of civil rights activist Maya Angelou to young women: "Life's a bitch. You've got to go out and kick ass."

On that note, when you claim your rightful place, people may call *you* "bitch."

Consider throwing back what Tina Fey said on *Saturday Night Live*: "Bitches get stuff done."

Shift the Environment

Years ago, I spent a few months in Mexico and Guatemala, living with local families and studying Spanish in areas where few spoke English. It takes a lot more cognitive flexibility to adapt to such circumstances than a week at Club Med Cancun, where lack of ability to *hablar español* matters not.

Not that there is anything wrong with Club Med. My kids love the trapeze.

A land built upon immigration is one rich in creativity. That's because immigrants go through a major environmental and cultural shift when moving to a new land with different languages and customs and laws. A 2009 study published in the *Journal of Personality and Social Psychology* examined the link between multiculturalism and creative thinking. The researchers found that those who lived abroad had significant boosts in their ability to have sudden aha moments, where an idea "leaps into consciousness." The authors list numerous examples of creative geniuses—Nabokov, Hemingway, Yeats, Picasso, Handel, Stravinsky, and others—who created many of their greatest works while living in foreign countries.

A bit of traveling doesn't do it, the study found. To challenge the brain to a new way of living, one needs to be immersed in this new environment as a resident. Maybe you *do* need to pack up your shit and head off somewhere for an *Eat Pray Love* experience.

Or perhaps not. This book already helped end one marriage among my beta readers, and I don't want a reputation as a home-wrecker. In this case, she'd been mistreated and betrayed, and reading the draft of *The Holy Sh!t*

Moment helped her have her own aha that it was time to end it and move away.

But environmental shift does speak to changing your surroundings to spark change. It's more chaos theory: change the initial conditions and see what new outcomes result.

A study by researchers at Harvard and Dartmouth Universities collected stories of both successful and failed life change from 119 people. It should not be surprising to learn that the successful ones were more likely to have had intense emotional experiences, external threats (fear of loss), and "focal events that often culminated in crystallizations of discontent." Conversely, the stories of failure were more likely to involve use of willpower and an interest in maintaining the status quo.

The types of change ran the gamut: career, education, relationships, addiction, health behaviors, and attitude toward life. Those who failed to change were able to cope: even though things were bad, they either weren't bad enough to crystallize discontent, or these people were good at tolerating bullshit. The changers had reached a breaking point; the final straw lay upon the dromedary's vertebrae.

An interesting aspect of successful change was the environmental shift.

Some had to switch jobs, education tracks, even countries to solidify the change. To drive home the power of environment, the study referenced veterans of the Vietnam War who were addicted to heroin while in country but found quitting easy upon returning home due to "dramatic change in the social milieu." New environments, new beginnings, new experiences can create new identities. And new identity, you'll recall, is a big part of this. Unleashing the true self and the values you hold dear are what makes change feel like destiny instead of drudgery.

Battling addiction can involve avoiding harmful social influences and cues. That's an important task for changing initial conditions, because it's difficult to initiate sudden change when the behavior you wish to alter is reinforced by the surrounding environment.

Professor Benjamin Gardner, whom I conversed with regarding the identity shift associated with pregnancy, mentioned *The Biggest Loser*, a "reality" television program I have long been critical of. It ran for seventeen seasons; on the show, people with significant obesity tried to lose as much weight as possible as fast as possible, vying for a large cash prize.

Stories abound of how most contestants on the show rapidly regained the weight. Some of it was due to the ridiculous way they lost weight in the first place and the negative effect on metabolic rate. But a lot of it had to do with environment.

"On *The Biggest Loser,* they change behaviors but not habits," Professor Gardner said. "It's because of a new situation." They were taken out of their homes and placed into a high-pressure labor camp on a starvation diet; this stopped habits from translating into action. After they left the show, they returned home to their usual cues and triggers, and reverted to previous behaviors, regaining the weight.

Not all, however. Some kept the weight off because celebrity altered their identities. It doesn't justify the show's horrible existence, but some used the experience of becoming public figures to make a career of health and fitness, wherein part of who they became focused on keeping the weight off.

Wendy Wood, a professor of psychology at the University of Southern California, referenced the dramatic drop in smoking rates over the past few decades to reveal how environmental shifts lead to behavior change. "You can't smoke in your workplace," she said. Also, "Advertising is removed at point of purchase. You have to remember the exact brand and ask for it." She refers to these as examples of "friction" in the environment that make it difficult to continue an undesirable behavior. Gas-cap tethers and over-size diesel nozzles are other sources of friction: they help prevent you from doing the wrong thing.

Wood says the environment can help or hinder. For some, they feel trapped. They can't afford to leave a job or a relationship and get stuck. This is an unfortunate reality, but there are ways to alter one's surroundings and create an environment conducive to an enlightening experience.

Kounios and Beeman suggest creating "a sense of psychological distance, and a promotion orientation."

Recall how being active outside in an expansive environment enhances function of the prefrontal cortex, promoting creative thought. Kounios and

Beeman explain that this broadens attention rather than constrains it, because "static surroundings encourage static thinking." Conversely, "Enforced change and adaptation will destabilize entrenched thoughts through fixation forgetting to lubricate your mind for breakthrough ideas."

Far out.

Change routines in as many ways as practical, or even not that practical. Rearrange your workplace or furniture, even if it freaks out the dog. Start taking walks outside, heading in new directions, and vary the time of day. Interact with different people, go to different places, read unusual articles and books, play a new game, try a new sport, try yoga, try *anything*, as long as it's different.

Go on a quest to create chaos in your life, in bits and pieces or a fell swoop. Let the thoughts such disruptions engender meander and collide. Couple this with your other tasks of working on problems until you get stuck, then engage in distraction. Await your epiphany while also getting on with your life and endeavoring to meet the *poof* partway.

ACT Accordingly

Despite this *not* being a weight-loss book, there has been ample discussion of adding physical activity. Because it's good for you and has those awesome spillover effects into other areas of life.

Say you want to begin exercising but haven't yet. You're driving home from a dogshit day at the office, tired and frustrated, and want to become one with the couch like a stoner with a bag of Cheetos and a Netflix subscription. On the drive home, you see someone jogging down the street. Inspiring, right?

Yeah, no.

Seeing that person can make you *less* inclined to exercise because it creates cognitive dissonance: mental discomfort from having your actions be out of line with your beliefs. You believe you *should* be exercising, but you're not. And since you aren't yet willing to change your actions, you instead change your beliefs to alleviate the discomfort. In this case, you might make excuses about both you and the jogger you saw. You may imagine, hypothetically, that they have a lot of free time, while your schedule is harried. It makes you feel better by inventing this excuse.

It's not logical, but we do it. The question is, What do we do about it?

Acceptance and commitment therapy (ACT) can help. It involves mindfulness practice to get in touch with the present moment and realize what you're doing. If you see the jogger and invent that scenario, endeavor to stop and catch yourself in the act. Don't judge it or label it, just become aware and accept the reality of the situation.

Then, ask a question: *Who do I want to be in this moment?*

Do you want to be a person who scoffs at the jogger, imagining all this free time they have, or do you want to consider your own reasons for change, and perhaps commit to just five minutes to see how it goes?

It doesn't always work, which is why it's called mindfulness "practice." There will be times when it is easy to catch yourself and make the right choice, and other times, not. But such practice can pay off. A 2015 study of thirty-nine sedentary women by researchers at McGill University in Montreal found such interventions got people exercising harder, perceiving less exertion, and enjoying it more.

ACT alone isn't going to cause epiphany lightning to strike, but it's all part of the opening of one's mind to new experience, as well as a useful tactic in meeting the *poof* partway. Professor Nathan DeWall has some advice in this regard, as he had a life-changing epiphany about running but drove the habit home using his knowledge of the science of self-control to reach a lofty goal that few on the planet ever achieve.

I introduced Nathan in chapter 3 while examining the science of spillover effect; his life changed in April 2011, when his mother fell in her driveway and hit her head. It started a brain bleed, and she was airlifted to a hospital in Lincoln, Nebraska. Nathan spent the next three nights at her bedside, but she never woke up.

She was only sixty.

"She was that one person in my life, other than my wife, that when things would happen, good or bad, she was the one I would reach out to." At her funeral, Nathan noticed people weren't talking about what she accomplished via her work, but rather spoke of the activities that gave her life meaning. "The experience shaped me," he said. "I realized my priorities were out of whack."

All his focus had been on his career as a professor of psychology. Beyond that, there was little he did that gave his life meaning. He sunk into a profound grief over the loss of his mother. He couldn't sleep; his health suffered.

A year later he joined a weight-loss program as a show of support for his wife and was surprised to learn he was classified as having obesity. The quantitative data prompted him to take beginner steps to get healthier, exercising a little and making changes to his eating habits. As part of the change, he tried running short distances. After two weeks of it, he was still in the infancy stages, then the lightning bolt struck.

"I can remember exactly where I was," Nathan said. "It is a flashbulb memory for me." It was August 2012, and he was sitting in his living room chair. His wife had checked some books out from the library, and on a whim, Nathan picked up *Eat & Run* by champion ultramarathon runner Scott Jurek; another person I've interviewed, but that's not important, I just like name-dropping. (Cameron Diaz says hi.)

Sitting in his chair, Nathan read Jurek's words about running the Western States 100-mile Endurance Run and the Badwater 135. "I remember thinking, *I can't believe he actually did this.*"

Then he saw Jurek's next words in the book, which changed his life: "Sometimes you just do things."

Sometimes you just do things. If that's not a good description for sudden inspiration, I'm not sure what is. And in the case of Nathan DeWall, reading those words hit him hard.

As he read the book he wondered about running a hundred miles, but with those five words he became committed in an instant. "At that moment, I said, 'I can do this. I *will* be doing this.'" Even though he'd only been running for two weeks, he never considered failing. DeWall didn't care what he had to do. "The train had left the station. It wasn't up for discussion."

Nathan described that lightning strike as critical, but one doesn't decide to run a hundred miles, then later complete the Badwater 135, on spark alone. For such lofty goals, he put System 2 and his knowledge of the psychology of behavior change to work.

"Self-control has three main ingredients," he explained:

1. Monitoring: This involves keeping track of thoughts, feelings, and actions. It has never been easier to do this with apps that can be downloaded onto your phone.
2. Standards: It is necessary to pick a specific goal, like Nathan with running one hundred miles.
3. Strength: When you start something new, it will hurt and take a lot of energy, but over time you get stronger. "Some of the most exhilarating times are early on," DeWall said, "because you get big gains right away."

Monitoring and standards, DeWall explained, create a positive feedback loop. They keep motivation to continue the high via little hits of dopamine. And working on improving strength—reaching any goal, physical or not, requires this—provides the ability to attain it.

A year after Nathan began running, he was in Hell.

That's Hell, Michigan, the starting line of his first hundred-mile race. Four years later, he completed the Badwater 135.

Regarding the sudden death of his mother and his own declining health that resulted, "There is a lot to be said for the power of negativity in a person's life," he said. "People don't say, 'I was feeling so good I decided to change my life.'" Crystallization of discontent opens the doorway to endless possibility.

To quote the thirteenth-century Persian poet Rumi: "The wound is the place where the Light enters you."

Meditating toward the Magic Moment

I meditate all the time. I just happen to be lifting heavy things when I do it.

Don't quote me on that. It wasn't me. It was some buff bro who is too cool for meditation, seen on Facebook. I have a lot of those guys on my friend list, it seems. The irony of iron is, lifting requires intense concentration. I love it, but it's the opposite of letting your mind wander; if you do that, a barbell may end up crushing your trachea because you were pondering your purpose during a bench press.

How can meditation help induce a life-changing epiphany? It begins with a wee bit o' chillin' dafuq out.

We've covered a lot of the reasons why this is important. There is hitting rock bottom. There is not being happy, feeling like you're in a hole and seeking a way out. Life is less than awesome, or swirling the drain, or somewhere in between. Peak discontent is near, but there is no flash of inspiration, because anxiety triggers the opposite brain state required for epiphany.

Relaxation, mindfulness, and a positive mood while in a distracted state—where thoughts are permitted to meander and collide—are what allow the unconscious mind to merge with the conscious and let the anterior cingulate neuro-google *The Answer*.

There is a scientific journal with the name *Psychoneuroendocrinology*. I want you to lay back, get comfortable, close your eyes, and chant "psycho-neuroendocrinology" over and over as your mantra. Not really. I bring it up because of a 2016 study published in that journal about using meditation to reduce stress responses via self-compassion meditation. Did you know they can test your spit to find out how stressed you are? When your sympathetic nervous system goes down, which is indicative of a less stressed state, it can be measured by a reduction in salivary alpha amylase. There's another possible mantra for you to chant: "salivary alpha amylase."

They also checked anxiety responses to stress tests and found "robust effects on buffering stress" in the 105 test subjects. And it was just a short bit of meditation: a ten-minute audio recording to help them relax. Speaking of which, if you decide you want to delve into self-compassion meditation, having an audio guide can be beneficial. I can only do so much via the written word to guide you through meditation, so I'll recommend the website of Kristin Neff, an associate professor of psychology at the University of Texas at Austin, and an expert in self-compassion-oriented meditation. At self-compassion.org there are several free guided meditations under the "Practices" tab.

I listened to the "Self-Compassion/Loving-Kindness Meditation" audio clip. Here are some highlights:

- Get comfortable, settle into how your body feels, be in your body and fully inhabit it.
- Allow your attention to move outward to what sounds are around you. Don't reach out to them; let them arrive.
- Focus on your breathing, simple and easy; feel your chest rise and fall.
- Notice peacefulness of being quiet, just resting.
- Bring to mind a mistake or failure that's been bothering you. Try to get in touch with your feelings about it. Are you sad? Isolated? Inadequate?
- How does thinking about it make you feel? Does it create a tightness in your throat or a heaviness in your heart?
- Get in touch with the suffering caused by fear of not being good enough.
- Place one or two hands gently over your heart in a soft and comforting manner. See if you can let your heart be moved by how difficult the emotional experience is of thinking about this thing that makes you feel bad about yourself.
- Understand you are an imperfect being, just like everyone else. We all make mistakes. Repeat these silently to yourself: May I be safe. May I be peaceful. May I be kind to myself. May I accept myself as I am. Repeat a couple of times and reach for the intention behind the words.

That's an encapsulation of the first half of a twenty-minute guided meditation. If you feel like there is benefit for you, visit Professor Neff's site and have a listen. Alternatively, there are plenty of other meditation resources and apps you can find via a quick search.

One of them is from actress Carrie-Anne Moss.

Despite Hollywood pressures, she said she's not motivated by vanity, but self-care. "Self-care is so much more than a beauty regimen or an external thing you do," Moss told me. "It has to start within your heart to know what you need to navigate your life. A pedicure doesn't last, but meditating every day does." She said meditation has "created the most radical shift in my ability to handle stress and show up to take care of other people."

Those "other people" in her life include a husband and three young children.

Moss says she was "transformed" by motherhood; it's a higher priority to her than battling evil machines in *The Matrix* or assisting a troubled superhero named *Jessica Jones*. Meditation, she says, allows her to connect more deeply with her family by gaining personal insight and deciding who she wants to be in any specific moment.

Moss became so passionate in exploring the benefits of self-care she started a company, working with relevant experts, called Annapurna Living (annapurnaliving.com) that offers online courses on meditation, motherhood, and living in the moment.

Carrie-Anne's meditative approach is more about internal than external transformation. "You might still be doing the same job, but you infuse it with this connection with yourself," she said. "All of a sudden you realize what is important to you because you're no longer on the hamster wheel. If we just stop and connect to the truth of who we are we can stop running around in circles."

And yet, some people don't like the calm voice walking them through meditation and would rather just . . . walk.

It helps if you add some meditation to that stroll.

A 2017 study published in the *American Journal of Health Promotion* examined the effects on anxiety of walking coupled with meditation in 110 young adults. In addition to a control group, they had a walking-only group, a meditate-then-walk group, and a walk-then-meditate group. Walking by itself didn't do much to reduce anxiety, but meditation alone did. Meditation plus walking also worked well, but the study showed meditation was the key ingredient.

But that's just looking at anxiety. We know walking outside spurs creative thought. Numerous great thinkers throughout history have extolled the virtues of walking to enhance creativity. In fact, Aristotle founded the

Peripatetic School; translated from ancient Greek, it means "given to walking about," and legend has it the name came from Aristotle's penchant for doing so while thinking and lecturing.

Nabokov and Thoreau extolled its virtues. Charles Dickens was known to take lengthy walks each day, and Nietzsche said, "All truly great thoughts are conceived while walking." Nobel Prize winner Daniel Kahneman writes, "I did the best thinking of my life on leisurely walks."

So, chill a bit using the meditative strategy of your choosing to get into a less anxious, more positive state, and go for a stroll. Just don't expect epiphany to happen on that first walk or the fifth. Or the tenth. And don't forget about "shower thoughts"—another environment ripe for sudden insight.

Patience remains key. In his 1933 book *The Use of Poetry and the Use of Criticism,* T. S. Eliot wrote of creativity needing a period of "incubation," and that "we do not know until the shell breaks what kind of egg we have been sitting on." He refers to such hatching as a "mystical experience," one that is "characterised by the sudden lifting of the burden of anxiety and fear which presses upon our daily life so steadily that we are unaware of it."

Solitude for Seeking Enlightenment

We've examined a variety of stories covering multiple holy-shit moments. In some cases, people were alone, in others, not. When in the presence of others, they sometimes played a role in triggering epiphany; either knowingly or not, they helped it along.

In the modern world, we have a problem with distraction and little time for solitude, little time to be alone with our thoughts. And your brain is finicky. The creative flow of imagination, rumination, the meandering and colliding of various bits of data stored in the different processing centers of your brain, can be derailed by someone talking, an explosion on TV, a radio DJ, or the ping of a text message.

The goal is to *broaden* your thinking; things that demand attention *narrow* it. In *The Eureka Factor,* the authors stress that remaining fixated on a personal problem doesn't help solve it. One more time: analyze until stuck, *then distract.* Distraction is when thinking can broaden, and it can take some time to let go of the chaos of focused thinking. "Perhaps the single most important thing to remember is that your mental states can change," the authors write, "but they can't turn on a dime." It's not easy to switch back and forth between System 1's insightful thinking and the analytical mind-set of System 2. Leaving aside social media and email for five minutes of peace, only to jump back online, doesn't usually cut it.

It helps if you consider that seemingly doing nothing with your mind is actually doing *something.*

In a 2010 piece for *Scientific American,* Dr. Marcus Raichle, a professor of radiology and neurology at Washington University School of Medicine in St. Louis, wrote about the brain's "dark energy." Dr. Raichle states, "A great deal of meaningful activity is occurring in the brain" when you're not actively using it. Rather, "Dispersed brain areas are chattering away to one another."

The brain at "rest," which can be daydreaming, is using almost as much energy as when your brain is performing a task such as reading. There is only about a 5 percent difference, and even then, that 5 percent increase is localized to the part of the brain being used to complete the task; the over-all increase in energy expenditure between a "resting" brain and one that is solving equations is minuscule. More fascinating is that 60–80 percent of the energy consumed by the brain "occurs in circuits unrelated to any external event." That's where the dark-energy analogy comes from: referring to the unseen energy comprising most of the universe.

Most of the brain is busy doing stuff we cannot fathom. The adult brain, Dr. Raichle told me, makes up only about 2 percent of a human's body weight, yet it accounts for more than 20 percent of the body's energy expenditure. No wonder my dreams are so weird.

Let's get back to walking for a moment. I wrote of how being active outdoors engenders "soft fascination." The environmental stimuli are emotionally positive, which we know is good for insight, because they *seduce* your attention rather than *demand* it.

However, Dr. Raichle explains, when "vigilance is required because of novel or unexpected sensory inputs," the internal chatter among the dispersed areas of the brain diminishes. And so the area in which you go for a walk can affect your degree of vigilance.

As much as living abroad was lauded earlier for its ability to expand the mind, it's ironic that philosopher Immanuel Kant, born in the small German city of Königsberg in 1724, lived there for seventy-nine years without ever traveling beyond the city limits. But he walked every day, in late afternoon, rain or shine, always taking the same route. His path through the park became known as the "Philosopher's Walk."

He walked alone.

Being alone, undistracted, no need for vigilance because his feet had traced this path many thousands of times, the dark energy of Kant's brain flowed, connecting various components to talk to one another and discover new and interesting things about time, space, thinking, and knowing. Immanuel Kant's most famous work, *Critique of Pure Reason,* has been referred to as "arguably the most significant single work in the history of modern philosophy."

Kant's unvarying routine may also contradict what was said earlier about walking in different directions at varying times of day. You may wish to try both. Perhaps Kant's method will work for you, or bipedal variety may suit better. So long as the environment isn't hyperstimulating, as it might be for a newbie in New York, I expect it will serve.

Speaking of avoiding stimulation, leave your phone at home. If you must have it in case of emergency, tuck it away on "do not disturb" mode. If you require further convincing, a 2014 study published by researchers at the University of Sussex and University College London found higher media multitasking leads to lower gray-matter density in the anterior cingulate cortex, a critical part of the brain for detecting weakly activated answers arising from the unconscious. That brain area is what helps you discover the epiphany, and your damn smartphone is strangling it. Conversely, it's worth noting that a 2011 Harvard Medical School study examined the brain effects of an eight-week long mindfulness meditation intervention and discovered it *increased* gray-matter density in the area adjacent to the anterior cingulate, the posterior cingulate cortex, as well as in the hippocampus—regions involved in memory, sense of self, empathy, and stress control. Such research reveals the plasticity of the adult brain; the structure and function of it can improve in response to training.

Alone time, perhaps while walking in a calming environment, allows the mind to wander and talk to itself to create novel solutions to unique problems. Coupled with meditation to reduce anxiety, it creates an improved, unfocused state where thinking is broadened to entertain multiple ideas.

Henry David Thoreau left society behind in 1845 to live in the woods alone for more than two years, during which he wrote some of his greatest works. That seems extreme and likely not practical for your life. More reasonably, Einstein was a noted daydreamer who accomplished great things while remaining part of society. After months of intense mathematical study, he had his breakthrough on special relativity while taking a rest and letting his mind wander.

That's how it works.

Your Perfect Storm

"You are searching your environment for things that might coalesce into the perfect storm," Professor Ken Resnicow told me. It's not just gathering information, but gathering stimuli, getting as much raw material in place as you can in any old weird way. Thinking new thoughts using different methods, broadening your mindscape and letting the various bits of gray matter talk to one another. Whether it be quitting an addiction, starting an exercise regimen, launching a new career, starting a new relationship, or fixing an old one, there are a thousand different inspirations and motivations to do it, explains Resnicow. And so each individual, passionately driven epiphany will be a unique recipe that creates the storm.

Gather the bits of information. Process them using the methods provided in this book. And "have faith they will one day coalesce," Resnicow said. "Your storm is coming."

Your storm is coming.

Act Now!

- Beware the status quo bias; avoid adopting a "yeah, whatever" approach to doing things, and nudge yourself out of being mired in a mediocre life.
- To expose the greatness lying within, commit to overcoming fear via development of competence and confidence. Courage comes from action.
- Break your programming. Realize how society foists roles upon you for things to do and be; reject those constraints to open a world of freedom and possibility beyond what is considered "normal."
- Consider environmental shifts, either big or small. It can be as little as rearranging furniture or as big as moving to another country—or anywhere in between. Change forces your mind to expand in new directions.
- If bad habits need breaking, seek ways to create friction between the habit and the behavior. Create metaphorical gas-cap tethers and larger diesel nozzles you can use to stop you from doing something you know you don't want to do.
- Try cool new shit. Visit new places, meet new people, play at new things, read new books and articles. Embrace chaos and expand your mind, remembering that it all serves to "destabilize entrenched thoughts" so you can "lubricate your mind for breakthrough."
- When you find yourself changing your thoughts by making excuses to battle cognitive bias, try to catch yourself. Don't judge it but become aware and accept reality. Then ask yourself: *Who do I want to be in this moment?*
- For lofty, specific goals (like running one hundred miles), create the three main ingredients of self-control: monitoring, standards, and strength.
- Remember that anxiety triggers analysis, whereas a positive mood enables insight. Use meditative techniques to relax and

let anxiety slip away, putting your mind in a better state to achieve epiphany.

- Consider the site self-compassion.org for meditative guides, or search online or an app store for a tool that suits your personality best.
- Walk outside! You can do it in a chaotic manner, varying time and place, or be more like Immanuel Kant and make it always the same. Pick the way that lets your thoughts feel most free to meander and collide. Don't forget to couple with a bit of meditation beforehand to relax the mind into a positive state.
- Shower thoughts!
- Seek solitude to be alone with your thoughts, away from the distraction of devices and other people. Leave the phone at home or put it on "do not disturb" mode.
- Keep collecting and analyzing data. Be patient and retain faith that one day it will all coalesce. Your storm is coming.

10

SHAMANS, DRUGS, AND ROCK AND ROLL: EXTERNAL ASSISTANCE IN THE REEVALUATION OF REALITY

What a long strange trip it's been.
—JERRY GARCIA

On a fall day in 2013, I was engaged in fatherly duties, taxiing children to some critical appointment or another, radio set on the alternative rock station—the one we could all agree on. It has a "No Nickelback Guarantee."

Lorde finished singing "Royals," and a commercial came on: "Only nine days left to get tickets to the see *MythBusters* 'Behind the Myths' tour—"

Hell broke loose.

My son had been watching the show since it first aired when he was only five, captivated by their proclivity for blowing shit up. My daughter, who is three years younger, eventually joined him in his viewing when she tired of that sniveling shitbag *Caillou*. A decade later, *MythBusters* was by far their favorite show. Adam and Jamie were their heroes.

"You have to get us tickets to the show!" they cried in unison. "You have to interview them, and get us tickets up close, and get us backstage passes!"

[activates sarcasm] "Sure," I said. "No problem."

Cue more freaking out.

I said I would try, and damn if I didn't pull it all off. One of my editors said, "I love the *MythBusters*!" and she green-lit the article. Adam and Jamie were game, the publicist gave us tickets for the middle of row 9, and I even got the kids backstage passes for the meet-and-greet after the show.

For one day, I was a cool dad.

Backstage, my son told Adam how *MythBusters* inspired him to become an engineer. Adam was most encouraging.

Four years later, my son had just finished his first year of engineering school, his GPA near perfect.

Isn't that a cute story?

This next story of "young man dreams of being an engineer" has less of a *Chicken Soup for the Soul* vibe.

He was an acquaintance, years ago, and he told me how after finishing high school, he lacked direction and was working a dead-end job. One night, he got baked on hallucinogenic mushrooms and went to a party. A couple of guys from his old school were there. They'd just finished their first year of engineering. The two young men were animated in their discussion of how much they loved their classes and their professors and the experiments they conducted. Listening intently, and quite likely influenced by the drugs, a window in his mind opened. In an instant, he knew he too had to become an engineer. Suddenly, it was his *vision*.

He registered for classes. He got his degree. He had a successful career and was well thought of by those who worked with him.

"I love that story!" proclaimed James Fadiman when I told him. Fadiman has a Ph.D. in psychology from Stanford University and is an authority on the use of psychedelic drugs for transformative experiences.

Before we go further, a public service announcement:

OBEY THE LAW!

Also, understand that little is known regarding long-term effects of things like LSD (aka "acid") and psilocybin (aka "magic mushrooms"). Anecdotal claims are prevalent, and "microdosing" is a hot thing, but there is almost no quality research from the last half century studying safety or efficacy of such substances. Obey the law. Don't risk your health. The drug information in this chapter is provided for "far out, man" entertainment purposes only, and should *not* be taken as a recommendation.

Okay. Ass covered. Let's continue.

Elephant-Size Balls

Before The Man decided to be a real downer and classify these drugs as, like, super illegal, there was research into their use for treatment of psychiatric disorders and as therapies developed for battling alcohol addiction.

Fadiman told me stories of how, in the 1950s and 1960s, LSD was administered to hard-core drinkers as a last-ditch effort to get them clean. It began in the province of Saskatchewan. At the time, it was believed that alcoholics had to experience "rock bottom" to quit drinking. The concept: administering a mega dose of LSD would initiate the same kind of bad trip delirium tremens does (when people hallucinate from alcohol withdrawal, seeing spiders and snakes and shit), and frighten them into getting clean.

Except that's not what happened.

A typical "recreational" dose of LSD (lysergic acid diethylamide) is around 100 micrograms. Treatment for alcoholics was more than four times that, between 400 and 600 micrograms. The intent was to get these people to trip an elephant-size set of balls by taking a "transcendental dose." I asked Fadiman if this was a "guided trip," with a counselor talking them through it, but he said it was more like having a "babysitter."

There was little preparation, no instructions. The participants knew they were problem alcoholics and that this was another form of treatment, but that was it. They lay on a bed, wearing eyeshades and listening to music via headphones, and the "supervisor" was there to answer questions, hold their hands if they needed it, get them drinks of water. "It's a support function," Fadiman said. "They weren't diving into the person's psyche and thrashing around."

The results of early research were astounding. A 1955 study conducted at University Hospital in Saskatoon of twenty-four hard-core alcoholics using these methods saw six swear off alcohol completely, and another six drastically reduced their drinking and were able to obtain employment and reconnect with families. This is in line with Fadiman's claim of a 50 percent success rate, which, if true, blows away most other treatment methods.

Since we're on the subject, I'll repeat: Sudden cessation of drinking by the alcohol-dependent can be dangerous. If that's you, regardless of what inspires you to quit, consult a physician.

Lysergic Acid and the Long Term

A 2012 meta-analysis published in the journal *Psychopharmacology* examined six randomized controlled trials, comprising 536 participants, of old studies on the use of LSD for the treatment of alcoholism. The analysis proclaimed LSD therapy had "significant beneficial effect on alcohol misuse," but saw a fading of efficacy by the twelve-month period, suggesting repeated LSD therapy could be beneficial. James Fadiman was involved in numerous government-sanctioned LSD treatments in the 1960s in an outpatient clinic in Menlo Park near Stanford University. Some of the patients had been remanded by the court to undergo such therapy to treat their alcoholism.

Fadiman contests the study's claim regarding long-term efficacy, saying one treatment was usually enough.

How does it work? We're uncertain, but it wasn't the "freak the shit out of them with spiders and snakes" bad trip originally surmised. Fadiman explained that many who underwent treatment would then go out and drink and return and say one of two things: "What did you do to me?" or "I don't like drinking now." Fadiman said treatment hadn't removed the *physiological* enjoyment of alcohol, but it changed their psychology. "Your awareness becomes larger," he said. "People described it as seeing the universe is made of love."

Okay.

It has nothing to do with willpower, he explained, but a simple loss of interest in drinking. The things in their life making them desire obliteration no longer held meaning once they gained this new connection to the universe and themselves. In a 1969 study of 176 male alcoholics undergoing LSD treatment, published in *The American Journal of Psychiatry*, the researchers stated, "It was rather common for patients to claim significant insights into their problems, to feel that they had been given a new lease on life." Fadiman explained it being akin to a religious experience, except without the religion.

Speaking of hallucinogenic drugs, religion, and alcoholism, the story of Alcoholics Anonymous cofounder Bill Wilson bears investigation. Deep into detoxification from alcohol, he had a religious epiphany, where he felt a "Presence" and "a great peace." Then he said, "It burst upon me that I was a free man."

There is more to Bill's tale of sudden renouncing of alcohol. Dude was tripping.

In 1934, after several failed attempts to quit, Wilson staggered into Towns Hospital for substance abuse in New York City. He was first sedated with chloral hydrate and paraldehyde to calm his agitation from detoxing, allowing him to sleep. He was regularly wakened to be administered a cocktail that included tincture of belladonna, a potentially toxic plant that can cause hallucinations.

On the second or third day of detox, Mr. Wilson's former drinking buddy, Ebby Thacher, visited him. Thacher had gotten clean from alcohol by embracing Christianity and implored Wilson to turn himself over to Jesus to be liberated from addiction. The hallucinations that belladonna engender tend to be based on recent discussions, made fantastical. Wilson called out, "If there be a God, let him show himself!" He saw a blinding light, felt peace, and that was it. He never drank again.

James Fadiman explained the power of the hallucinogenic trip to battle alcohol addiction as a fundamental identity change. "The person who is rewarded by excessive alcohol consumption no longer exists." Those parts of the personality are "transcended."

Regarding psilocybin, Fadiman says the difference between it and LSD in terms of "life-changing potential and intensity, is zero." They are identical, except LSD lasts about twice as long, as much as twelve hours. I asked him about the mushroom trip of my old acquaintance, who became an engineer after hearing about the program from former classmates, and Fadiman surmised, "He was able to truly get into their emotional mental space. Listening to a couple of guys saying they like their work doesn't change someone's life, but if you can feel how they feel about it, then it can."

A Rich History of Hallucinating

In chapter 6, the use of peyote was examined as part of the ceremonies of the Native American Church. Fadiman says the primary active ingredient in peyote is mescaline, which "is interchangeable with LSD and psilocybin. The effects are fairly similar."

In 1994, Sandor Iron Rope explained, the American Indian Religious Freedom Act was amended to allow for Native Americans to legally use peyote for religious and other purposes.

However, peyote is far from the only psychoactive substance used for attaining religious insight. The planet is filled with countless varieties of naturally occurring hallucinogens used by various peoples for centuries. These are referred to as "entheogens," a combination of two ancient Greek words coined in 1979 by ethnobotanists to mean "that which causes God to be within an individual." They have psychoactive properties and are used for spiritual purposes. Throughout history, and on every continent except Antarctica (as hilarious as hallucinating penguins might be; hey, that's going to be my band name: the Hallucinating Penguins), there are examples of shamanic usage of such substances for achieving spiritual insight. Mushrooms, root barks, hashish, mandrake, henbane, kava, and many other entheogens across the ages have been used to induce visions, reach higher understanding.

I'm not recommending you begin randomly eating plants and licking cane toads to have an epiphany. But it's interesting to understand the rich history of the quest for insight. Since the dawn of humanity, we've been seeking answers to the questions of our lives.

I hope this book helps you find yours.

High on Dark Energy

I'll end this final chapter with my own (strange) story.

In the introduction, I mentioned using some of these methods to make the ground shift for myself, initiating massive and effortless change. I was in the preliminary stages of investigating life-changing epiphany, knowing far less than I (and you) do now, but I stumbled my way forward. I'll be damned if it didn't work.

I quit drinking.

The thought of never drinking again seems . . . boring. I *like* alcohol. I've had good times with beer in hand. When I decided to quit, I knew it wasn't forever.

I chose to stop for a year.

I didn't have a Problem, or a *problem,* but perhaps a wee "problem." For thirty years, I drank on the wrong side of moderate. However, I also eat healthy and exercise lots, both of which provide a partial "get of out jail free" card when it comes to negative consequences of ethanol indulgence.

Alcohol wasn't running me down, yet. Life was good; very good. I figured without drinking, it could be great.

With my first epiphany—the Joan Baez one—even though it transformed my life, it only had a modest impact on my drinking. Since then, I had tried and failed to cut down many times. Any effort at reducing intake never lasted more than a few weeks. Stress drinking was common. I've been floor-licking drunk more times than I can remember.

I read a few stories of people taking a year off, and my visceral reaction was always, "Fuck that." FYI, that's the sole F-bomb in this book. I saved it to relay how strongly opposed I was to the idea of not drinking for a year. That attitude changed, quickly, on the day before Christmas 2015.

I was out for a run. It was a beautiful, sunny day, not too cold. The snow was hard-packed, not slippery. I was excited for the next day's celebrations. Everything was ready: all the food purchased, the presents wrapped, plenty of booze. I was looking forward to my annual Christmas day piss-up, where I prepare a feast for over a dozen family and friends and get royally fucked up in the process.

Okay. Two F-bombs.

Sudden insight struck: *the anticipation of inebriation does not reflect the true meaning of Christmas.* This revelation made taking a year off alcohol suddenly seem like a good idea, but more was needed to drive it home. I had to work for this epiphany via weird thoughts.

I had read research, conducted interviews, and written articles about epiphany already; I knew a few things. I knew sudden change was more about feeling than thinking. I'd read Plato's description of the charioteer, and Haidt's elephant-and-rider analogy. While pondering that, I realized I'd always considered less (or no) drinking from a *rational* perspective, mostly evaluating health risks (alcohol is a Group 1 carcinogen). I'd never wondered how I *felt* about potential benefits of change.

Inside a mere moment, I realized: *it's time.* Emotionally, not rationally, I was accepting of this idea because of the promise of something new. That was sudden insight number two. Yet I was still not all the way ready. I needed to think through a few more things first. Systems 1 and 2 engaged in a neurological dance.

With the charioteer, there are two horses representing emotion, but they are not like-minded. One is more virtuous in its passions; the other has baser appetites. While I see merit in simplifying down to one quadruped in the form of an elephant, I had a pair of battling *equi* to contend with.

I examined abstinence with positivity. As an adult, I'd never lived sober; I didn't know what it was like. This was an opportunity to discover a new way of living. Alas, there was pushback from the dark horse on the emotional-driver team. My ambition to become a better person (good horse) conflicted with my desire to lay in a beer-filled bathtub, scarfing potato chips and watching HD porn (bad horse).

I slowed to a walk. The two horses entered a rapid negotiation process; I had that booze at home, waiting to be drunk. I could have made the snap decision to start my year off right then—people do that all the time and are often successful—but there were a couple of events in January that the bad horse wanted to drink during.

An accommodation was reached. I'd drink on Christmas and during those special events in January, but otherwise not at all. Then, on February 1, I'd quit for a minimum of a year.

The imaginary door to this new, alcohol-free year lay open before me. It had been present since the first moment I realized taking a year off was a good idea, but it was now more crystallized via the efforts of System 2. It beckoned, but I could have turned away. I might have said, "Nah!" Soon after, I would have forgotten the door ever appeared.

I recalled the way I felt about it moments before: *it's time.* But there was still fear. I became aware that the air surrounding me felt like I was shrouded in fog. My life, with its regular imbibing and occasional overdrinking, was coated in a slightly noxious substance that no longer felt right. Ahead, through the door, there was clear, blue sky. The fog was known and, until moments earlier, comfortable. Forward was uncertain but held promise. The fog pulled at me with its tendrils, preventing me from advancing. To make the leap would require effort. There were important *insights* gained, but a final, transformative *sensation* was needed for the final push.

If I made this move, it would be without looking back. My desire for change had to be stronger than my fear. *Desire.* It was key. But how to make it *overwhelming*?

This is where we take a departure from science. To make the final step, I had to embrace chaos, change initial conditions, do something I'd never done.

Supertramp's "Even in the Quietest Moments" played on my iPod. Roughly 90 percent of rock songs are about someone the writer used to bang, is currently banging, or hopes to bang. Another 5 percent involve Hobbits or Vikings. Occasionally, however, lyricists compose something more philosophical, and it seemed to me Roger Hodgson was singing of his struggle to find communion with a higher power. Maybe. Like with everything, including the shape of the earth, there is internet debate on the subject. But whatever, because in that moment, that's what the song spoke to me.

I was not raised in a religious home. I never had a faith and still don't. I respect the rights of others to believe as they wish, but the existence of God is something I'm more comfortable not worrying over. Nevertheless, part of me wondered if seeking otherworldly assistance might not be a method of enhancing motivation.

I enjoy science fiction; it doesn't mean I know jackshit about astrophysics. This is about a temporary personal hypothesis to achieve a goal, not scientific veracity. Recall from the previous chapter the mention of dark energy; it makes up approximately 68 percent of the stuff of the universe. NASA has some ideas, but states, "More is unknown than is known" about it. And so, for a moment, I envisioned such energy as a kind of *Star Wars*–like "Force" I could access to power myself forward.

For lack of a better word, I "prayed" to the universe to lend me strength. I speculated on the subatomic potentiality lurking in the deepness of space, waiting to be utilized if only the appropriate conduit for expression were available. I fantasized about opening a rift in the Space-James Continuum, reaching through to that energy source and, as Yoda said, "letting the Force flow."

And suddenly, I was infused. Face flushed, arms and legs tingling, the cells of my body electrified.

Was it paranormal? I am most skeptical. I consider it more a self-induced neurochemical cascade achieved via a meditative state. A person can have a similarly powerful emotional sensation by watching the end of *Marley & Me*. It doesn't mean God did it.

Whatever it was, it lit up my brain in a new way. Then serendipity lent a hand in the choice of the next song.

Awash in a rush of happy hormones, I heard George Ezra asking me over and over what I was waiting for. At last, possessing the power to move forward, I awakened to the reality that I was done waiting. The last piece fell into place; a snap decision was made. It was time to use the Force, Luke.

In that instant, I approached the imaginary door and stepped out of the fog and into a clear new day.

It was that abrupt mental movement forward that made the change real. My mind shifted in a split second from mere pondering, to absolute certainty. *Elation!* I began running again with renewed vigor.

There was no challenge, nothing to resist. Part of my identity transformed into one of curiosity of what total abstinence would be like. I approached it with a sense of adventure. During that time I traveled to Europe and South America, twice visited Vegas, skied and saw concerts; not once did I desire a drop.

I kept going when the year was up. After seventeen months of no alcohol, I had my forty-ninth birthday in New York, having just finished a series of meetings with publishers for this book. I met a friend for lunch at a pub named P. J. Clarke's in Midtown; I had fish tacos washed down with two pints to celebrate.

I didn't finish the second pint.

Over a year has passed since then. There is no longing. My intake is less than a quarter what it was prior to the hiatus. On Christmas Day 2017—historically my drunkest day of the year—I had three drinks. New Year's Eve, I split a single drink with my wife.

I wrote about the benefits of quitting for the *Chicago Tribune,* managing to sneak in talk of harder erections in a family newspaper. I was less stressed, stopped napping, and much to my and my wife's surprise, became far handier around the house.

I have many positive things in my life that don't involve alcohol. As much as I enjoyed drinking, life doesn't revolve around it. This tale is not meant to minimize the horror of addiction; not everyone can just snap out of it.

But because of my story, several did.

One was my mother; I told her the story of how I quit. For fifty years, she'd been hitting the red wine pretty hard, likely connected to her horrible childhood. Like me, she'd tried and failed to cut back many times. But my tale resonated, and she suddenly quit. Mom says she's done for good, and she hasn't had a drop for two years, saying she doesn't miss it.

Another is Coryn Samaras Griffeth of Annapolis, Maryland.

Ten months after quitting, I published a post describing the epiphany I generated to break from alcohol. Coryn read it. The next day, she quit, too.

Coryn had started drinking when she was twelve. Even though she went to Princeton, which she described as "super lame—not a party college at all," she was a big drinker in college. "Two nights a week I got shit-faced."

She kept up her partying ways after school finished, taking a break for having children, then got back at it. Now in her forties, she describes a couple of defining moments that prompted her to quit. In mid-November 2016, "I hosted a dinner party for friends I really respected, and just got annihilated. I was so embarrassed the next day. It wasn't cute anymore. It was just sad."

Two weeks later, she read my article about taking a year off. It resonated, it got her thinking; she mentioned it to her husband. But that night, she got drunk again on cheap wine and blew chunks.

The next morning, November 27, her first conscious thought upon waking was, *I'm done.* "I knew it right away when I woke up," she said. "I told my husband, 'I'm done for a year.'"

She had no doubts, it wasn't difficult. And it was a good year. She enjoyed "being completely present at all times, feeling more mentally sharp and efficient. There were no more wasted days." Coryn went beyond the year by an extra month, having two glasses of champagne on New Year's Eve. She said the desire to drink is gone, and she has no plans to drink again soon.

Self-Service

I'm not writing an "Act Now!" section for this chapter. I don't want anyone thinking I recommend taking illegal and/or unregulated drugs to induce epiphany. Instead, I'll finish with something certain to appear self-serving.

People say I'm good at this.

Over the years, I've received countless messages about how something I wrote or said suddenly changed a life. And yet, what happened with this book surprised me. I had several beta readers for the first draft. I was seeking both general and specific feedback prior to submitting to my editor, Elizabeth Beier, at St. Martin's Press.

I was looking for comments on the jokes, writing style, science, grammar, structure. . . . "Dude, you talk about poop *way* too much."

From most, that's not the feedback I got.

"Dude, I had an epiphany reading this book," the majority said.

I chose my beta readers for their knowledge of psychology, religion, writing, and editing experience. I didn't think, *This person really needs this book.* But epiphanies happened anyway.

Cool, right?

I hope this will generate belief *in* you and *for* you. Some may be skeptical reading that a book can change a life, but it happens. If you believe that, believe *this* book can help inspire you to live your best life. Believe in the words of Helen Keller: "Optimism is the faith that leads to achievement. Nothing can be done without hope and confidence."

Have hope. Have confidence. It doesn't matter where positive life change comes from.

So long as it comes.

THE LOVE WE FOUND

I came alive. I could fly.

—CHARLIE PARKER

harles Dickens's *A Christmas Carol* is the tale of how the wealthy must be supernaturally terrorized into sharing. It's still a nice story; my family has a tradition of watching the Muppet version each Christmas Eve. "Light the lamp, not the rat!"

In my reading of the phenomenon of epiphany, the experience of Ebenezer Scrooge was mentioned several times, but he's not the best example of a life-changing flash of insight. Because it wasn't a flash. It took the better part of a night, various realizations, and *three* ghosts to fully bring him around. Were it a true epiphany, I expect one ghost would suffice.

You want to talk sudden, Christmas Day epiphany? Look no further than *The Grinch.* "Maybe Christmas, he thought . . . doesn't come from a store. Maybe Christmas, perhaps . . . means a little bit more!"

Then, in a moment, his heart grew three sizes, which in the literal, modern medical world, is generally lethal. But in Dr. Seuss's story it imbued amazing strength. Ol' Grinch had a sudden realization based on a new bit of information—Christmas doesn't come from a store. It coalesced stuff in his brain, and he changed, just like that, then took inspired action.

That's what happened to me with reading "Action is the antidote to despair." It was a simple and new bit of information that was extraordinarily relevant and important to me at that space in time. It had profound impact on my thought processes moving forward as a fundamental truth to follow for the rest of my life. Baez's words are a form of mantra for me. I remember them when things go wrong. They give me strength.

But such strength can come at a cost.

This book involves digging into your psyche; you may find scary stuff if you go deep enough. What's more, things you take pleasure in today you could end up forgoing in favor of the new you. Because it *is* a new you coming to the fore. Sudden and massive life change isn't about willpower or habit formation, but a shift in identity and values. Just because the new identity arrives quickly doesn't mean it's always a painless process, this exposing of the true self, this ceding of control.

Quick and easy. I've railed against it for years, calling it bullshit. And it mostly is. To achieve greatness, there is much work, but inspiration can arrive quickly, making the work destiny rather than drudgery. So, not easy, but . . . *resolved.* And excited. The quest becomes imperative; it will keep you awake when you should sleep. "Easy" isn't the right word.

There may be emotional turmoil ahead, but love finds a way.

At the end of *The Muppet Christmas Carol,* there is a song titled "The Love We Found." (Who knew Michael Caine had a passable singing voice?) This is what life-altering epiphany is about: love is found.

Think of key words I've written to describe it: *rightness, destiny, vision, compelling, passion, desire, undeniable, excited, determined.* . . . Plus, you know, that whole chapter titled "The Power of Love."

Love can make your heart grow three sizes in a single day, figuratively, imparting great strength.

You can come to desire more from life and more from yourself, as well as want to make the world a better place. You can't love everyone. Humanity is sometimes a dick sandwich that's tweeting on Ambien. But if more of us are inspired to drag the people-train forward, it will result in fewer dicks.

That's my wish for humanity: fewer dicks.

Wil Wheaton, formerly Wesley Crusher of *Star Trek: The Next Generation,* has a simple philosophy of living: "Don't be a dick." It's great advice, but *you* can aspire to more. You can be a beacon. You can accomplish great things if inspired, and serve not only your own needs and interests, but lift others up, too.

You can create a world with fewer dicks.

Michelle Obama said, "Success isn't about how much money you make, it's about the difference you make in people's lives."

Do you want to remain mired in mediocrity, or is there desire to let the dog off the chain, the grizzly out of the cage, the horse past the gate? Tiptoe safely to death? *Screw that.* Make a difference in people's lives, yours included.

Epiphanies changed my life for the *much* better. Sudden, overwhelming inspiration took me from half-assed to "Hell, yeah!" Countless others have had the same amazing experience. I want you to feel it, too, that incredible sensation when your life is divided into "before" and "after." You realize things will never be the same and rejoice at the revelation.

Poet Mark Anthony wrote: "And one day she discovered that she was fierce, and strong, and full of fire, and that not even she could hold herself back because her passion burned brighter than her fears."

That could be you.

We have but one run at this life; make it a good one.

Sir Winston Churchill died January 24, 1965, age ninety. He got first quote in this book; I wish to give him last word as well. And they were his last recorded words. My final inspirational advice is asking you to ponder your deathbed, which I hope is many years from now. Imagine being able to say this as your goodbye:

"It has been a grand journey—well worth making once."

ACKNOWLEDGMENTS

"Class, for this project, you'll be forming teams of . . ."

Ugh. It was always death. I hated team projects in school. As an adult, however, I learned the more good people you have on your team, the better work you create. And I have had so many good people to help me write this book. Amazing people.

My agent, Peter Steinberg at Foundry Literary + Media, gets first mention because he had so much influence on the direction I took in writing it. Can you believe this book was almost written in a serious tone without a single mention of poop? Peter encouraged me to embrace my regular, silly voice and forget trying to be someone I'm not. He also asked me to investigate the "how to" angle, which was the greatest of ideas. And he got me the book deal. That part is important, too. Yfat Reiss Gendell, the cofounder of Foundry, was helpful in pushing me to come up with a unique idea. I'm in debt for her suggestion that I read Malcolm Gladwell. It was doing so that primed my mind for sudden insight into how I should approach this topic.

When I walked out of the offices of St. Martin's Press in the Flatiron Building in downtown New York, I said to Peter, "I hope she makes an offer. I like her."

"Her" is Elizabeth Beier, executive editor for St. Martin's. She said,

"You're a funny writer" in the meeting, which always melts my heart. The first draft I submitted was much different from the book you hold in your hands. I like to think I know good advice when I hear it, and Elizabeth's recommendations on how to improve *The Holy Sh!t Moment* were excellent. During every conversation I found myself nodding and saying, "I love that idea." The entire team at St. Martin's has been helpful and a joy to work with. I also wish to thank freelance copy editor Kate Davis for her meticulous eye.

Steven M. Ledbetter, a behavior-change consultant and CEO of Habitry (habitry.com), spent a number of hours on the phone with me in the early stages of this book as an expert advisor, giving me greater insight into the psychology of behavior change and suggesting experts to interview. I was delighted when he approved of what I'd created.

I also want to thank Alan Levinovitz, an assistant professor of religious studies at James Madison University, for his insights and suggestions for improving the chapter on religious epiphanies.

Carrie King, Martha Mantikoski, Sarah Deveau, Kris South, Natalia Reagan, Scott Stratten, and Kris Huiberts—thanks, all of you, for reading the early versions and for your feedback to help make it better.

Thank you to the people who follow and interact on my Facebook page. Reading many thousands of comments about your hopes, dreams, trials, tribulations, victories, defeats, feelings, experiences, insights, advice, and feedback have shaped my writing in ways beyond measure.

Thanks Craig McArthur for taking me skiing when I needed a break. Thanks Rob Sawyer for the mentoring and ongoing encouragement. Thanks to my amazing children for the writing material and for mostly listening when I said I needed quiet to work on edits. Thanks to my mom and two dads for all their love and support over the years.

And thank you, Heidi, my most wonderful wife, for reasons too numerous to mention.

NOTES

Introduction: *The Librarian Who Put Down the Cigarettes and Picked Up a Sword*

11 A 2011 study published: Betsy Sparrow et al., "Google Effects on Memory: Cognitive Consequences of Having Information at Our Fingertips," *Science* 333 (2011): 776–78.

12 a 2014 study published: Michelle Eskrit and Sierra Ma, "Intentional Forgetting: Note-Taking as a Naturalistic Example," *Memory & Cognition* 42 (2014): 237–46.

15 From the ancient Greek: From https://en.wikipedia.org/wiki/Epiphany (feeling) (retrieved November 25, 2015).

16 In his book *The Myths*: Scott Berkun, *The Myths of Innovation* (Newton, MA: O'Reilly Media, 2010), 9.

17 "When you tackle a: John Kounios and Mark Beeman, *The Eureka Factor* (New York: Random House, 2015), 102, 109.

18 It's a parameter of: Albert Bandura, "Self-Efficacy: Toward a Unifying Theory of Behavioral Change," *Psychological Review* 84 (1977): 191–215.

1. The Antidote to Despair: The Euphoria of the Life-Changing Moment

26 The concept began with: Plato, *Phaedrus*, trans. Benjamin Jowett, http://classics.mit .edu/Plato/phaedrus.html (retrieved May 4, 2017).

27 The allegory was adapted: Jonathan Haidt, *The Happiness Hypothesis: Finding Modern Truth in Ancient Wisdom* (New York: Basic Books, 2006).

27 A short time later: Chip Heath and Dan Heath, *Switch: How to Change Things When Change Is Hard* (Toronto: Random House Canada, 2010), 8.

29 In *The Eureka Factor*: John Kounios and Mark Beeman, *The Eureka Factor* (New York: Random House, 2015), 7.

30   Kahneman refers to this: Daniel Kahneman, *Thinking, Fast and Slow* (Toronto: Anchor Canada, 2013), 20–21.

30   the supporting character: Ibid., 31, 35.

30   Kahneman says System 1: Ibid., 58.

30   It is a "mental shotgun": Ibid., 99.

30   A 2011 study published: Rainer Greifeneder et al., "When Do People Rely on Effective and Cognitive Feelings in Judgment?," *Personality and Social Psychology Review* 15 (2011): 107–41.

33   meta-analysis of twenty-seven: Jennifer Di Noia and James Prochaska, "Dietary Stages of Change and Decisional Balance: A Meta-Analytic Review," *American Journal of Health Behavior* 34 (2010): 618–32.

35   William Miller and his: William Miller and Janet C'de Baca, *Quantum Change* (New York: Guilford Press, 2001), 8.

36   Of the fifty-five people: Ibid., 14, 23.

37   In 2016, researchers from: Elliot Berkman et al., "Finding the 'Self' in Self-Regulation: The Identity-Value Model," *Psychological Inquiry* 28 (2017): 77–98.

40   This is called the: Martin Fishbein, "Attitude and the Prediction of Behaviour," in *Readings in Attitude Theory and Measurement,* ed. Martin Fishbein (New York: Wiley, 1967).

42   In a 2013 study: Angelina Sutin and Antonio Terracciano, "Perceived Weight Discrimination and Obesity," *PLOS ONE* 8 (2013): epub.

42   And a 2003 study: Kristin Neff, "Self-Compassion: An Alternative Conceptualization of a Healthy Attitude Toward Oneself," *Self and Identity* 2 (2003): 85–101.

49   "One does not become": Rollo May, foreword to *Existential-Phenomenological Alternatives for Psychology*, by Ronald S. Valle and Mark King (Oxford: Oxford University Press, 1978).

49   In his 1950 book: Rollo May, *The Meaning of Anxiety* (New York: Ronald Press, 1950).

51   chaos theory has been: Ian Stewart, *Does God Play Dice?* (Cambridge, MA: Blackwell, 1989).

2. Embracing Chaos: Quantum vs. Linear Behavior Change in the Role of Epiphany

62   A 2016 Nielsen report: *The Nielsen Total Audience Report,* Q4, 2016, 10.

64   An example of how: Stuart Ferguson et al., "Unplanned Quit Attempts—Results from a U.S. Sample of Smokers and Ex-Smokers, *Nicotine & Tobacco Research* 11 (2009): 827–32.

64   A 2005 study published: Morgen Kelly et al., "Sudden Gains in Cognitive Behavioral Treatment for Depression: When Do They Occur and Do They Matter?," *Behavioural Research and Therapy* 43 (2005): 703–14.

65   In 1998, a study: Roy Baumeister et al., "Ego Depletion: Is the Active Self a Limited Resource?," *Journal of Personality and Social Psychology* 74 (1998): 1252–65.

66   Researchers from Curtin University: Martin Hagger and Nikos Chatzisarantis, "A

Multilab Preregistered Replication of the Ego-Depletion Effect," *Perspectives on Psychological Science* 11 (2016): 546–73.

66 A 2007 study published: Timothy Carey et al., "Psychological Change from the Inside Looking Out: A Qualitative Investigation," *Counselling & Psychotherapy Research* 7 (2007): 178–87.

67 On the same day: Susan Dominus, "When the Revolution Came for Amy Cuddy," *New York Times,* October 18, 2017, https://www.nytimes.com/2017/10/18/magazine /when-the-revolution-came-for-amy-cuddy.html (retrieved October 18, 2017); Joe Simmons and Uri Simonsohn, "Power Posing: The Evidence Behind the Most Popular TED Talk," *Data Colada*, May 8, 2015, http://datacolada.org/37 (retrieved May 25, 2018).

67 The 2016 study of: Elliot Berkman et al., "Finding the 'Self' in Self-Regulation: The Identity-Value Model," *Psychological Inquiry* 28 (2017): 77–98.

67 And a 2017 study: Katharina Bernecker et al., "Implicit Theories about Willpower Predict Subjective Well-Being," *Journal of Personality* 85 (2017): 136–50.

68 Can you pump up: Vanessa Allom et al., "Does Inhibitory Control Training Improve Health Behaviour? A Meta-Analysis," *Health Psychology Review* 10 (2016): 168–86.

68 More disconcerting is a: Eleanor Miles et al., "Does Self-Control Improve with Practice? Evidence from a Six-Week Training Program," *Journal of Experimental Psychology* 45 (2016): 1075–91.

68 Inzlicht coauthored a 2017: Marina Milyavskaya and Michael Inzlicht, "What's So Great About Self-Control? Examining the Importance of Effortful Self-Control and Temptation in Predicting Real-Life Depletion and Goal Attainment," *Social Psychological and Personality Science* 8 (2017): 603–11.

68 A 2012 study published: Vanessa Patrick and Henrik Hagtvedt, "'I Don't' Versus 'I Can't': When Empowered Refusal Motivates Goal-Directed Behavior," *Journal of Consumer Research* 39 (2012): epub.

68 A 2015 study of: Gregory Miller et al., "Self-Control Forecasts Better Psychosocial Outcomes but Faster Epigenetic Aging in Low-SES Youth," *Psychological and Cognitive Sciences* 112 (2015): 10325–30. For additional studies on the negative health impacts of enforced self-control, see G. H. Brody et al., "Is Resilience Only Skin Deep? Rural African Americans' Socioeconomic Status-Related Risk and Competence in Preadolescence and Psychosocial Adjustment and Allostatic Load at Age 19," *Psychological Sciences* 24 (2013): 1285–93; E. Chen et al., "Neighborhood Poverty, College Attendance, and Diverging Profiles of Substance Use and Allostatic Load in Rural African American Youth," *Clinical Psychological Science* 3 (2015): 675–85.

69 Nevertheless, William Miller: William Miller, "The Phenomenon of Quantum Change," *Journal of Clinical Psychology* 60 (2004): 453–60.

70 but in *Quantum Change*: William Miller and Janet C'de Baca, *Quantum Change* (New York: Guilford Press, 2001), 21–22.

70 This particular illusion first: Esther Inglis-Arkell, "The World's Most Famous—and Ambiguous—Illusion," October 16, 2014, https://io9.gizmodo.com/the-worlds-most -famous-and-ambiguous-illusion-1646895274 (retrieved November 22, 2017).

70 *Gestalt* is a German: Sam Atkinson and Sarah Tomley, eds., *The Psychology Book* (New York: DK Publishing, 2012), 44.

71 In *The Eureka Factor*: John Kounios and Mark Beeman, *The Eureka Factor* (New York: Random House, 2015), 5.

74 Janet C'de Baca, a clinical: Janet C'de Baca and Paula Wilbourne, "Quantum Change: Ten Years Later," *Journal of Clinical Psychology* 60, no. 5 (2004): 531–41.

74 It likely wasn't Einstein: Alice Calaprice, ed., *The Ultimate Quotable Einstein* (Princeton, NJ: Princeton University Press, 2010), 474.

74 Instead, the quote appears: Narcotics Anonymous pamphlet, 1981, 11, https://web .archive.org/web/20121202030403/http://www.anonymifoundation.org/uploads /NA_Approval_Form_Scan.pdf (retrieved February 21, 2018).

76 In 2008, he had: Kenneth Resnicow and Scott Page, "Embracing Chaos and Complexity: A Quantum Change for Public Health," *American Journal of Public Health* 98 (2008): 1382–89.

78 has published research about: Ruth Ann Atchley et al., "Creativity in the Wild: Improving Creative Reasoning through Immersion in Natural Settings," *PLOS ONE* 7 (2012): epub.

3. You, Part 2: Finding Purpose via Epiphany

83 In *The Eureka Factor*: John Kounios and Mark Beeman, *The Eureka Factor* (New York: Random House, 2015), 10.

84 "Existence precedes essence": This comes from a lecture Jean-Paul Sartre delivered on October 29, 1945, at Club Maintenant in Paris. Titled "Existentialism Is a Humanism," it was first published by Nagel that year, then translated into English in 1948 by Philip Mairet and Carol Macomber; http://www.mrsmoser.com/uploads/8 /5/0/1/8501319/english_11_ib_-_no_exit_-_existentialism_is_a_humanism_ -_sartre.pdf (retrieved January 13, 2018).

84 Albert Camus, another French: "The Myth of Sisyphus" is a 1942 essay by Albert Camus, first published in English in 1955 by Hamish Hamilton, translated by Justin O'Brien, http://www2.hawaii.edu/~freeman/courses/phil360/16.%20Myth%20 of%20Sisyphus.pdf (retrieved January 13, 2018).

84 It's ancient Greek: *Nicomachean Ethics* was written by Aristotle in 350 BC. Translated by W. D. Ross, it is available via The Internet Classics Archive: http://classics .mit.edu/Aristotle/nicomachaen.mb.txt (retrieved January 13, 2018).

85 William Du Bois, a political: Sam Atkinson, ed., *The Philosophy Book* (New York: DK Publishing, 2011), 234.

85 I am myself and: José Ortega y Gasset, *Meditations on Quixote*, first published in 1914; English ed. (New York: W. W. Norton, 1961).

85 That being written, Ortega: Atkinson, *The Philosophy Book*, 242–43.

85 William James (also dead): "Biography, Chronology, and Photographs of William James," https://www.uky.edu/~eushe2/Pajares/jphotos.html (retrieved January 13, 2018).

85 When it comes to *what*: William James, *The Varieties of Religious Experience* (Cambridge, MA: Harvard University Press, 1902).

85 James was also considered: "Biography, Chronology, and Photographs of William James."

86 In *Quantum Change,* Miller: William Miller and Janet C'de Baca, *Quantum Change* (New York: Guilford Press, 2001), 156–74.

86 Social psychologist Roy Baumeister: Roy Baumeister, "The Crystallization of Discontent in the Process of Major Life Change," in *Can Personality Change?*, ed. Todd Heatherton and Joel Weinberger (Washington, DC: American Psychological Association, 1994), 282, 287, 290.

87 In relation to epiphany: Miller and C'de Baca, *Quantum Change,* 162–64.

87 In her book *Mindfulness*: Ellen Langer, *Mindfulness,* 25th anniv. ed. (Boston: Da Capo Press, 2014), 48.

87 At his trial for: Plato, *Apology,* trans. Benjamin Jowett, http://classics.mit.edu/Plato /apology.html (retrieved January 13, 2018).

87 Søren Kierkegaard, a: Søren Kierkegaard, *The Sickness Unto Death,* first published in 1849, rev. ed., trans. Howard and Edna Hong (Princeton, NJ: Princeton University Press, 1983).

87 Twentieth-century German psychoanalyst: Karen Horney, *Neurosis and Human Growth* (New York: W. W. Norton, 1950), 64–85.

89 In 1979, Daniel Kahneman: Daniel Kahneman and Amos Tversky, "Prospect Theory: An Analysis of Decision Under Risk," *Econometrica* 47 (1979): 263–92.

89 A 2016 study published: Mitesh Patel et al., "Framing Financial Incentives to Increase Physical Activity Among Overweight and Obese Adults: A Randomized, Controlled Trial," *Annals of Internal Medicine* 164 (2016): 385–94.

90 which Kahneman expanded upon: Daniel Kahneman, *Thinking, Fast and Slow* (Toronto: Anchor Canada, 2013), 288.

90 which Kahneman referred to: Ibid., 412.

90 gave an apt example: Cass Sunstein, "Nudging Smokers," *New England Journal of Medicine* 372 (2015): 2150–51.

91 In 2014, Harvard University: Francesca Gino et al., "The Burden of Guilt: Heavy Backpacks, Light Snacks, and Enhanced Morality, *Journal of Experimental Psychology* 143 (2014): 414–24.

91 A pile of research: Inge Seiffge-Krenke and Nicolai Klessinger, "Long-Term Effects of Avoidant Coping on Adolescents' Depressive Symptoms," *Journal of Youth and Adolescence* 29 (2000): 617–30; A. Baitar et al., "The Influence of Coping Strategies on Subsequent Well-Being in Older Patients with Cancer: A Comparison with 2 Control Groups," *Psychooncology* 21 (2017): epub; J. W. Aarts et al., "The Relation between Depression, Coping and Health Locus of Control: Differences between Older and Younger Patients, with and without Cancer," *Psychooncology* 24 (2015): 950–57; C. Vigano et al., "Unrevealed Depression Involves Dysfunctional Coping Strategies in Crohn's Disease Patients in Clinical Remission," *Gastroenterology Research and Practice* 8 (2016): epub; L. Muller and E. Spitz, "Multidimensional Assessment of

Coping: Validation of the Brief Cope Among French Population," *L'Encephale* 29 (2003): 507–18; S. Jeavons et al., "Coping Style and Psychological Trauma after Road Accidents," *Psychology, Health & Medicine* 5 (2000): 213–21; M. S. Hagger et al., "The Common Sense Model of Self-Regulation: Meta-Analysis and Test of a Process Model," *Psychological Bulletin* 143 (2017): 1117–54; M. Perreault et al., "Employment Status and Mental Health: Mediating Roles of Social Support and Coping Strategies," *Psychiatric Quarterly* 18 (2017): 501–14; N. Sanguanklin et al., "Job Strain and Psychological Distress Among Employed Pregnant Thai Women: Role of Social Support and Coping Strategies," *Archives of Women's Mental Health* 17 (2014): 317–26.

91 Negative emotions are evolutionarily: Tori Rodriguez, "Negative Emotions Are Key to Well-Being," *Scientific American,* May 1, 2013, https://www.scientificamerican.com/article/negative-emotions-key-well-being (retrieved Nov 28, 2017).

92 That one is right: Abraham Maslow, "A Theory of Human Motivation," *Psychological Review* 50 (1943): 370–96.

92 You are not a blank: Abraham Maslow, *The Farther Reaches of Human Nature* (New York: Viking, 1971), 53.

92 It's worth noting that: Abraham Maslow, *Toward a Psychology of Being* (New York: Van Nostrand, 1968), 97–102.

93 Gabriele Oettingen cautions in: Gabriele Oettingen, *Rethinking Positive Thinking* (New York: Current, 2014), 34.

93 Oettingen asserts that: fantasizing: Ibid., 35–36.

94 "Passion has no expiration": Scott Barry Kaufman and Carolyn Gregoire, *Wired to Create* (New York: Tarcher Perigee, 2015), 16–18.

94 In her book, *The*: Gretchen Rubin, *The Happiness Project* (Toronto: Harper Collins, 2012), 11.

94 but Scott Kaufman countered: Kaufman and Gregoire, *Wired to Create*, 24–26.

95 In 2008, the two: Edward Deci and Richard Ryan, "Hedonia, Eudaimonia, and Well-Being: An Introduction," *Journal of Happiness Studies* 9 (2006): 1–11.

96 SDT is about the: Curt Lox et al., *The Psychology of Exercise* (Scottsdale, AZ: Holcomb Hathaway, 2010), 65–66.

97 in the same 2008: Richard Ryan et al., "Living Well: A Self-Determination Theory Perspective On Eudaimonia," *Journal of Happiness Studies* 9 (2008) 139–70.

98 The Rubicon metaphor relates: Kennon Sheldon et al., "Rightly Crossing the Rubicon: Evaluating Goal Self-Concordance Prior to Selection Helps People Choose More Intrinsic Goals," *Journal of Personality*, under review.

99 Winston was a soldier: James Humes, *The Wit & Wisdom of Winston Churchill* (New York: Harper Collins, 1994), xvi–xvii.

100 Collins opens *Good to*: Jim Collins, *Good to Great* (New York: Harper Business, 2001), 1.

100 Gallup's 2017 *State of*: Ed O'Boyle and Annamarie Mann, "American Workplace Changing at a Dizzying Pace," February 15, 2017, http://news.gallup.com/businessjournal/203957/american-workplace-changing-dizzying-pace.aspx (retrieved January 13, 2018).

100 William James asserted we: William James, *The Philosophy of William James* (New York: Modern Library, 1953).

100 Langer published a: Ellen Langer and A. Benevento, "Self-Induced Dependence," *Journal of Personality and Social Psychology* 36 (1978): 886–93.

101 as the Heath brothers: Chip Heath and Dan Heath, *Switch: How to Change Things When Change Is Hard* (Toronto: Random House Canada, 2010), 163.

101 A 2006 study by: V. Griskevicius et al., "Going Along Versus Going Alone: When Fundamental Motives Facilitate Strategic (Non)Conformity," *Journal of Personality and Social Psychology* 9 (2006): 281–94.

101 "Facts are better than": Collins, *Good to Great,* 69, 73–77.

102 Another tip from Collins: Ibid., 87.

102 Taking this a step: Ibid., 95–96.

102 When we find our: Ibid., 116.

102 The book reaffirms much: Ibid., 195–204.

102 I'll wrap up my: Ibid., 209.

105 Her first marathon was: Kathrine Switzer: Marathon Woman, "Accomplished Athlete," http://kathrineswitzer.com/runner/accomplishments/ (retrieved Nov 30, 2017).

107 DeWall referenced a study: Thomas Denson et al., "Self-Control Training Decreases Aggression in Response to Provocation in Aggressive Individuals," *Journal of Research in Personality* 45 (2011): 252–56.

108 Pulitzer Prize–winning investigative: Charles Duhigg, *The Power of Habit* (Toronto: Anchor Canada, 2014), 97–126.

108 I've often extolled the: Over years writing for the *Los Angeles Times* and *Chicago Tribune,* I've covered the myriad benefits of exercise. These columns feature interviews with respected experts and peer-reviewed research. A sampling includes: "Dumbbells Can Make You Brainy," *Los Angeles Times*, February 13, 2012; "Sweating Off the Sadness," *Chicago Tribune,* December 5, 2013; "Survivorcise," *Chicago Tribune,* September 26, 2012; "Exercise: Alternative Reward for those Battling Addiction," *Chicago Tribune,* June 12, 2013; "Training Your Brain for Creativity," *Chicago Tribune,* March 14, 2014; "Exercise Is the Best Medicine for Getting a Good Night's Sleep," *Chicago Tribune,* September 24, 2014; "Vanity Can Be a Healthy Asset," *Los Angeles Times,* August 22, 2011; "Go Ahead, Run into Old Age," *Los Angeles Times,* January 16, 2012; "Use Exercise to Squash Killer Stress," *Los Angeles Times,* August 8, 2011; "An Active Lifestyle Makes Life and Death Better," *Chicago Tribune,* March 6, 2015; "Outrun Diabetes," *Chicago Tribune,* November 1, 2012; "Taking Time Out for Exercise Pays in Spades," *Chicago Tribune,* August 25, 2012; "Make Your Money 'Work Out' for You," *Chicago Tribune,* June 20, 2012.

108 In self-determination theory: Lox et al., *The Psychology of Exercise,* 66.

109 From his 2004 study: William Miller, "The Phenomenon of Quantum Change," *Journal of Clinical Psychology* 60 (2004): 453–60.

4. What's Going On in There?: The Brain Science of the Holy Shit Moment

114 Just as I was: David Oakley and Peter Halligan, "Chasing the Rainbow: The Non-Conscious Nature of Being," *Frontiers in Psychology,* November 14, 2017.

115 Daniel Kahneman addressed this: Daniel Kahneman, *Thinking, Fast and Slow* (Toronto: Anchor Canada, 2013), 4.

115 A 2010 review article: in S. L. Bressler and V. Menon, "Large-Scale Brain Networks in Cognition: Emerging Methods and Principles," *Trends in Cognitive Sciences* 6 (2010): 277–90.

115 Researchers were examining the: L. Solomons and G. Stein, "Normal Motor Automatism," *Psychological Review* 3 (1896): 492–512.

115 That being said, Kounios: John Kounios and Mark Beeman, *The Eureka Factor* (New York: Random House, 2015), 99–101.

116 Mutual of Omaha launched: "Mutual of Omaha Announces America's Favorite Aha Moment," October 20, 2015, http://www.marketwired.com/press-release/mutual-of-omaha-announces-americas-favorite-aha-moment-2065358.htm (retrieved November 29, 2017).

116 A 2015 video compilation: "The Moment You Know," May 11, 2014, https://www.youtube.com/watch?v=DpI4n4N2_Yc&list=PLC8682D0463DE3074 (retrieved January 13, 2018).

118 What's fascinating is the: L. Hertz-Pannier et al., "Late Plasticity for Language in a Child's Non-Dominant Hemisphere: A Pre- and Post-Surgery fMRI Study," *Brain* 125 (2002): 361–72; D. Boatman et al., "Language Recovery after Left Hemispherectomy in Children with Late-Onset Seizures," *Annals of Neurology* 4 (1999): 579–86; F. Liegeois et al., "Language after Hemispherectomy in Childhood: Contributions from Memory and Intelligence," *Neuropsychologia* 46 (2008): 3101–7; F. Liegeois, "Speech and Oral Motor Profile after Childhood Hemispherectomy," *Brain Language* 114 (2010): 126–34.

118 Digging deeper into the: Kounios and Beeman, *The Eureka Factor*, 45.

118 In 2005, researchers at: Carlo Reverberi et al., "Better Without (Lateral) Frontal Cortex? Insight Problems Solved by Frontal Patients," *Brain* 128 (2005): 2882–90.

118 Kounios and Beeman assert: Kounios and Beeman, *The Eureka Factor*, 46.

118 Kounios and Beeman explain: Ibid., 37, 41, 43.

119 The anterior cingulate is: Ibid., 124.

120 For years prior to: John Kounios and Mark Beeman, "The *Aha!* Moment: The Cognitive Neuroscience of Insight," *Current Directions in Psychological Science* 18 (2009): 210–16; John Kounios and Mark Beeman, "The Cognitive Neuroscience of Insight," *Annual Review of Psychology* 65 (2014): 71–93; C. Salvi et al., "Sudden Insight Is Associated with Shutting Off Visual Inputs," *Psychonomic Bulletin and Review* 22 (2015): 1814–19; E. M. Bowden et al., "New Approaches to Demystifying Insight," *Trends in Cognitive Sciences* 9 (2005): 322–28; John Kounios et al., "The Prepared Mind: Neural Activity Prior to Problem Presentation Predicts Subsequent Solution by Sudden Insight," *Psychological Science* 17 (2006): 882–90; K. Subramaniam et al., "A Brain Mechanism for Facilitation of Insight by Positive Effect," *Journal of Cognitive Neuroscience* 21 (2009): 415–32; Mark Jung-Beeman et al., "Neural Activity When People Solve Verbal Problems with Insight," *PLOS Biology* 2 (2004): epub; John Kounios et al., "The Origins of Insight in Resting-State Brain Activity," *Neuropsycholo-*

gia 46 (2008): 281–91; J. I. Fleck, "The Transliminal Brain at Rest: Baseline EEG, Unusual Experiences, and Access to Unconscious Mental Activity," *Cortex* 44 (2008): 1353–63.

120 It provides temporal information: Kounios and Beeman, *The Eureka Factor*, 69.

120 Subjects were given the: Kounios and Beeman, "The *Aha!* Moment."

120 "We were amazed at: Kounios and Beeman, *The Eureka Factor,* 70.

121 Kounios and Beeman replicated: Ibid., 71.

121 At the moment of insight: Ibid., 84–86.

121 In a 2009 study: Kounios and Beeman, "The *Aha!* Moment."

122 That doesn't mean it's: Carey Morewedge and Daniel Kahneman, "Associate Processes in Intuitive Judgment," *Trends in Cognitive Sciences* 14 (2010): 435–40.

123 He referred to instinct: Sam Atkinson and Sarah Tomley, eds., *The Psychology Book* (New York: DK Publishing, 2012), 160–61.

123 prepared a report for: Leonid Perlovsky, *Neural Dynamic Logic of Consciousness: The Knowledge Instinct,* Report for the Airforce Research Laboratory, September 7, 2007.

124 This is reminiscent of: Immanuel Kant, *Critique of Pure Reason* (Cambridge, UK: Cambridge University Press, 1998), 50.

124 Kahneman refers to the: Kahneman, *Thinking, Fast and Slow,* 50.

125 The initial concept of: William James, *The Principles of Psychology* (New York: Henry Holt, 1890).

125 researcher Jonathan Evans: Jonathan Evans, "Dual-Processing Accounts of Reasoning, Judgment, and Social Cognition," *Annual Review of Psychology* 59 (2008): 255–78.

126 Eureka happened in a: Kounios and Beeman, *The Eureka Factor*, 27–28.

126 Scott Kaufman writes of: Scott Barry Kaufman and Carolyn Gregoire, *Wired to Create* (New York: Tarcher Perigee, 2015), 67.

127 Beeman and I spoke: Beyond the interview with Mark Beeman, there is additional information in Kounios and Beeman, *The Eureka Factor,* 22–23, and Bruce Weber, "Robert Sallee, Who Survived Smoke Jumping Disaster, Dies at 82," *The New York Times*, May 31, 2014, https://www.nytimes.com/2014/06/01/us/robert-sallee-survivor -of-smoke-jumpers-is-dead-at-82.html (retrieved May 26, 2018).

127 It turns out that: Kounios and Beeman, "The *Aha!* Moment." Also see chap. 9 of Kounios and Beeman, *The Eureka Factor.*

127 Kahneman echoes Kounios and: Kahneman, *Thinking, Fast and Slow,* 60.

128 In 2013, researchers from: Eddie Harmon-Jones et al., "Does Negative Affect Always Narrow and Positive Affect Always Broaden the Mind?: Considering the Influence of Motivational Intensity on Cognitive Scope," *Current Directions in Psychological Science* 22 (2013): 301–7.

128 In 2016, researchers from: Elliot Berkman et al., "Finding the 'Self' in Self-Regulation: The Identity-Value Model," *Psychological Inquiry* 28 (2017): 77–98.

128 research into people with: A. Bechara, et al., "Emotion, Decision-Making and the Orbitofrontal Cortex," *Cerebral Cortex* 10 (2000): 295–307; A. R. Damasio, "The Somatic Marker Hypothesis and the Possible Functions of the Prefrontal Cortex," *Biological Sciences* 29 (1996): 1413–20; A. Bechara and H. Damasio, "Decision-Making

and Addiction (Part I): Impaired Activation of Somatic States in Substance Dependent Individuals When Pondering Decisions with Negative Future Consequences," *Neuropsychologia* 40 (2002): 1675–89; A. Bechara et al., "Different Contributions of the Human Amygdala and Ventromedial Prefrontal Cortex to Decision-Making," *Journal of Neuroscience* 19 (1999): 5473–81; A. Bechara et al., "The Role of Amygdala in Decision-Making," *Annals of the New York Academy of Sciences* 985 (2003): 356–69; D. Tranel and A. Bechara, "Sex-Related Functional Asymmetry of the Amygdala: Preliminary Evidence Using a Case-Matched Lesion Approach," *Neurocase* 15 (2009), 217–34.

129 "Lose your mind and": Atkinson and Tomley, *The Psychology Book,* 117.

129 How to lose your: Kounios and Beeman, *The Eureka Factor,* 87, 90–91.

130 A 2011 study of: Mareike Wieth and Rose Zacks, "Time of Day Effects on Problem Solving: When the Non-Optimal is Optimal," *Thinking and Reasoning* 17 (2011): 387–401.

130 Loewi was a German: For more information on the story of Otto Loewi, see Alli McCoy and Yong Tan, "Otto Loewi (1873–1961): Dreamer and Nobel Laureate," *Singapore Medical Journal* 55 (2014): 3–4.

134 And study after study: Alan Delamater, "Improving Patient Adherence," *Clinical Diabetes* 24 (2006): 71–77; Leslie Martin et al., "The Challenge of Patient Adherence," *Therapeutics and Clinical Risk Management* 1 (2005): 189–99; J. Mata et al., "When Weight Management Lasts. Lower Perceived Rule Complexity Increases Adherence," *Appetite* 54 (2010): 37–43; L. E. Shay, "A Concept Analysis: Adherence and Weight Loss," *Nursing Forum* 43 (2008): 42–52; J. Mata and Todd Lippke, "Keep It On: How Complex Diet Rules Prevent Weight Loss," *Appetite* 50 (2008): 562.

135 DeYoung had a study: Colin DeYoung, "The Neuromodulator of Exploration: A Unifying Theory of the Role of Dopamine in Personality," *Frontiers in Human Neuroscience* 7 (2013): 762.

135 A 2000 study published: J. L. Monahan, "Subliminal Mere Exposure: Specific, General, and Diffuse Effects," *Psychological Science* 11 (2000): 462–66. For more information about mere exposure effect being adaptive in organisms, also see R. B. Zajonc, "Mere Exposure: A Gateway to the Subliminal," *Current Directions in Psychological Science* 10 (2001): 224–28.

136 In his book *The Power*: Charles Duhigg, *The Power of Habit* (Toronto: Anchor Canada, 2014), 112.

136 And a 2011 spotlight: Teresa Amabile and Steven Kramer, "The Power of Small Wins," *Harvard Business Review,* May 2011.

137 Mark Beeman told me: In addition to my interview with Professor Beeman, see Kounios and Beeman, *The Eureka Factor,* 21–22.

138 Folkman's sudden insight and: Diane Bielenberg and Patricia D'Amore, "Judah Folkman's Contribution to the Inhibition of Angiogenesis," *Lymphatic Research and Biology* 6 (2008): 203–7; Andrew Pollack, "F.D.A. Approves Cancer Drug from Genentech," *New York Times,* February 27, 2004, http://www.nytimes.com/2004/02/27/business/fda-approves-cancer-drug-from-genentech.html (retrieved January 1, 2018).

138 Albert Einstein said conceiving: Kounios and Beeman, *The Eureka Factor,* 125.

139 A 2010 study into: Sascha Topolinski and Rolf Reber, "Gaining Insight into the 'Aha' Experience," *Current Directions into Psychological Science* 19 (2010): 402–5.

139 first described by Hungarian: Mihaly Csikszentmihalyi and Jeanne Nakamura, "Effortless Attention in Everyday Life: A Systematic Phenomenology," in *Effortless Attention: A New Perspective in the Cognitive Science of Attention and Action,"* ed. Brian Bruya (Cambridge, MA: MIT Press, 2010), 181.

139 When professional jazz musicians: C. J. Limb and A. R. Braun, "Neural Substrates of Spontaneous Musical Performance: An fMRI Study of Jazz Improvisation," *PLOS ONE* 27 (2008): epub.

5. The Rock-Bottom Hypothesis: The Power of Epiphany to Battle Addiction

143 Ample research reveals the: I interviewed Jennifer Dewey, fitness director for Betty Ford, for "Exercise: Alternative Reward for those Battling Addiction," *Chicago Tribune,* June 12, 2013. For additional research on how exercise helps battle addiction, see David Raichlen et al., "Wired to Run: Exercise-Induced Endocannabinoid in Humans and Cursorial Mammals with Implications for the 'Runner's High,'" *Journal of Experimental Biology* 215 (2012): 1331–36; M. S. Buchowski et al., "Aerobic Exercise Training Reduces Cannabis Craving and Use in Non-Treatment Seeking Cannabis-Dependent Adults," *PLOS ONE* 6 (2011): epub; P. J. Gates et al., "Psychosocial Interventions for Cannabis Use Disorder," *Cochrane Database of Systemic Reviews* 5 (2016): epub; D. Wang et al., "Impact of Physical Exercise on Substance Use Disorders: A Meta-Analysis," *PLOS ONE* 9 (2014): epub; N. Siñol et al., "Effectiveness of Exercise as a Complementary Intervention in Addictions: A Review," *Adicciones* 25 (2013): 71–85; Mark Smith and Wendy Lynch, "Exercise as a Potential Treatment for Drug Abuse: Evidence from Preclinical Studies," *Frontiers in Psychiatry* 2 (2011): epub.

144 It's a story told: Chip Heath and Dan Heath, *Switch: How to Change Things When Change Is Hard* (Toronto: Random House Canada, 2010), 119–20.

144 a gas leak triggered: "Piper Alpha: How We Survived North Sea Disaster," BBC News, July 6, 2013, http://www.bbc.com/news/uk-scotland-22840445 (retrieved January 13, 2018).

144 Chip and Dan Heath: Heath and Heath, *Switch,* 120.

144 a 2005 study of: H. Matzger et al., "Reasons for Drinking Less and their Relationship to Sustained Remission from Problem Drinking," *Addiction* 100 (2005): 1637–46.

145 In her book, Langer: Ellen Langer, *Mindfulness,* 25th anniv. ed. (Boston: Da Capo Press, 2014), 181.

146 published in the *British*: Robert West and Taj Sohal, "'Catastrophic' Pathways to Smoking Cessation: Findings from National Survey," *British Medical Journal* 332 (2006): 458–60.

146 In Miller's book *Quantum*: William Miller and Janet C'de Baca, *Quantum Change* (New York: Guilford Press, 2001), 24–25.

148 One benefit of a: Ibid., 128–31.

148 Miller writes in *Quantum*: Ibid., 157.

148 researchers from the University: P. A. Linley and S. Joseph, "Positive Change Following Trauma and Adversity: A Review," *Journal of Traumatic Stress* 17 (2004): 11–21.

148 A more recent study: Ines Blix et al., "Posttraumatic Growth, Postraumatic Stress and Psychological Adjustment in the Aftermath of the 2011 Oslo Bombing Attack," *Health and Quality of Life Outcomes* 11 (2013): epub.

149 a 2016 review of: Margaret Westwater et al., "Sugar Addiction: The State of the Science," *European Journal of Nutrition* 55 (2016): epub.

149 in a 2014 article: J. Hebebrand et al., "'Eating Addiction,' Rather than 'Food Addiction,' Better Captures Addictive-Like Eating Behavior," *Neuroscience & Biobehavioral Reviews* 47 (2014): 295–306.

153 also the 2013 study: Ann Marie Roepke, "Gains Without Pains? Growth After Positive Events," *Journal of Positive Psychology* 8 (2013): 280–91.

6. The Hand of God: Exploring Religious Epiphany

156 On June 11, 1963: "Monk Suicide by Fire in Anti-Diem Protest," *New York Times,* June 11, 1963, https://vietnamandamericansociety.files.wordpress.com/2013/09/saigon-10.pdf (retrieved January 14, 2018).

156 President John F. Kennedy: Malcolm Brown, "The Self-Immolation of Thich Quang Duc in Saigon," *New Statesman,* April 1, 2010.

156 one of his autobiographies: Winston Churchill, *My Early Life: 1874–1904* (London: T. Butterworth, 1930).

158 case of James Arthur Ray: John Dougherty, "For Some Seeking Rebirth, Sweat Lodge was End," *New York Times,* October 21, 2009. See also, "Sweat Lodge Leader Sentenced to Two Years in Prison," CNN, https://www.cnn.com/2011/11/18/justice/arizona-sweat-lodge-sentencing/index.html (retrieved January 20, 2018).

159 In his book on: James Kellenberger, *Religious Epiphanies Across Traditions and Cultures* (New York: Palgrave Macmillan, 2017), 9.

159 William James wrote of: Sam Atkinson, ed. *The Philosophy Book* (New York: DK Publishing, 2011), 209.

159 Mohandas Gandhi had an: Rebecca Brown, "Perfecting Political Performance: Spinning and Gandhian Virtuosity," in *Political Aesthetics: Culture, Critique and the Everyday,* ed. Arundhati Virmani (London: Routledge, 2014), 140–41.

159 Martin Luther King, Jr.: John Dear, "The God at Dr. King's Kitchen Table," *National Catholic Reporter,* January 16, 2007, https://www.ncronline.org/blogs/road-peace/god-dr-kings-kitchen-table (retrieved December 8, 2017).

159 During a grave illness: Claudia Stokes, "The Mother Church: Mary Baker Eddy and the Practice of Sentimentalism," *The New England Quarterly,* September 2008, 438–61.

160 Bill Wilson called out: Alcoholics Anonymous, *Alcoholics Anonymous: The Story of How Many Thousands of Men and Women Have Recovered from Alcoholism* (New York: Alcoholics Anonymous World Services, 1976), 27.

160 And one of the most: Justin Holcomb, "The Five Solas-Points from the Past That Should Matter to You," https://www.christianity.com/church/church-history/the -five-solas-of-the-protestant-reformation.html (retrieved January 14, 2018); Angie Broks, "Martin Luther Too Had an Epiphany," https://medium.com/@angiebroks /martin-luther-too-had-an-epiphany-e36ccaade985 (retrieved January 14, 2018).

160 Miller and C'de Baca refer: William Miller and Janet C'de Baca, *Quantum Change* (New York: Guilford Press, 2001), 21–22.

161 William Miller reported this: Ibid., 24.

161 From the people Miller: Ibid., 30.

161 The researchers did notice: Ibid., 72–73.

162 A 2007 study of: S. E. Zemore, "A Role for Spiritual Change in the Benefits of 12-Step Involvement," *Alcoholism: Clinical & Experimental Research* 31 (2007): 76S–79S.

162 In a 2008 book: M. J. Pearce et al., "Spirituality and Health: Empirically Based Reflections on Recovery," *Recent Developments in Alcoholism* 18 (2008): 187–208.

166 It was the single: Miller and C'de Baca, *Quantum Change,* 30.

167 On the same page: Winston Churchill, *My Early Life.*

167 Doss was awarded the: The film *Hacksaw Ridge* was made after Doss rejected telling the tale over the years because he was unwilling to have parts of his story fictionalized. The Desmond Doss Council was formed and only gave rights to the story if it would remain true to the facts, which the film largely has done. One such example of a minor change is that Doss was not court-martialed, as was portrayed in the film, but rather was merely threatened with it by an officer. One part that was left out of the film as "hard to believe" was that, after having taken the brunt of a grenade explosion to save the lives of his comrades, Doss was being carried off the field by fellow soldiers while under heavy fire. Seeing another badly wounded man, Desmond rolled off the stretcher and crawled over to treat him. Doss then gave up his stretcher to the man. While Doss was waiting for help to come back, a Japanese sniper shot him, shattering his left arm. He made a splint out of the stock from a rifle and crawled three hundred yards to an aid station. In addition to my interview with his son, Desmond Doss, Jr., sources include Booton Herndon, *Redemption at Hacksaw Ridge* (Coldwater, MI: Remnant Publications, 2016 rerelease); the 2003 documentary film *The Conscientious Objector,* https:// www.youtube.com/watch?v=9vf7fbbwPr0 (retrieved February 22, 2018); "Desmond Doss: The Real Story," https://desmonddoss.com/bio/bio-real.php (retrieved February 22, 2018); "Frequently Asked Questions and Answers about Desmond T. Doss," https:// desmonddoss.com/hacksaw-ridge-movie/faq.php (retrieved February 22, 2018).

7. The Power of Love: How Passion for Life and Love Inspires Sudden Change

174 Carl Rogers married his: Sam Atkinson and Sarah Tomley, eds., *The Psychology Book* (New York: DK Publishing, 2012), 136.

175 He developed the concept: Carl R. Rogers, "Client-Centered Approach to Therapy," in *Psychotherapist's Casebook: Theory and Technique in Practice,* ed. I. L. Kutash and A. Wolf (San Francisco: Jossey-Bass, 1986).

175 Problems arise when we: Atkinson and Tomley, *The Psychology Book,* 134.

175 Love is the only: Viktor Frankl, *Man's Search for Meaning* (Boston, MA: Beacon Press, 1959).

177 A 2004 study published: Jens Förster et al., "Temporal Construal Effects on Abstract and Concrete Thinking: Consequences for Insight and Creative Cognition," *Journal of Personality and Social Psychology* 87 (2004): 177–89.

177 Five years later, the: Jens Förster et al., "Why Love Has Wings and Sex Has Not: How Reminders of Love and Sex Influence Creative and Analytic Thinking," *Personality and Social Psychology Bulletin* 35 (2009): 1479–91.

178 "Love is a bridge": Max Scheler "Love and Knowledge," in *On Feeling, Knowing, and Valuing: Selected Writings* (Chicago: University of Chicago Press, 1992), 152.

178 *Cogito ergo sum* is: René Descartes, *Discourse on the Method of Rightly Conducting One's Reason and Seeking Truth in the Sciences,* 1637, http://www.earlymoderntexts .com/assets/pdfs/descartes1637.pdf (retrieved January 14, 2018).

178 Max Scheler would disagree: Sam Atkinson, ed. *The Philosophy Book* (New York: DK Publishing, 2011), 240.

181 is a teachable moment: Ellinor Ollander et al., "Beyond the 'Teachable Moment'—A Conceptual Analysis of Women's Perinatal Behavior Change," *Women and Birth* 29 (2016): e67–71.

184 A 2017 study of: Jack Levin et al., "Are More People Disturbed by Dog or Human Suffering?" *Society and Animals* 25 (2016): 1–16.

184 A 2017 study by: Juliane Kaminski, "Human Attention Affects Facial Expressions in Domestic Dogs," *Scientific Reports* 7 (2017): epub.

184 One thing they might be trying: Peter F. Cook et al., "Awake Canine fMRI Predicts Dogs' Preference for Praise *vs* Food," *Social Cognitive and Affective Neuroscience* 11 (2016): 1853–62.

184 And if you have siblings: Samantha Deffler et al., "All My Children: The Roles of Semantic Category and Phonetic Similarity in the Misnaming of Familiar Individuals," *Memory & Cognition* 44 (2016): 989–99.

185 *The New York Times*: Mike McPhate, "California Today: The Stories That Moved Us in 2016," *New York Times,* December 30, 2016.

189 researchers at Manhattan College discovered: Katherine Jacobs Bao and George Schreer, "Pets and Happiness: Examining the Association between Pet Ownership and Wellbeing," *Anthrozoös* 29 (2016): epub.

8. Dreamers Aren't Doers: Making Positive Fantasies Work for You Instead of Against You

194 This is the first: William Miller and Janet C'de Baca, *Quantum Change* (New York: Guilford Press, 2001), 178–79; Roy Baumeister, "The Crystallization of Discontent in the Process of Major Life Change," in *Can Personality Change?* ed. Todd Heatherton and Joel Weinberger (Washington, DC: American Psychological Association, 1994), 287, 290.

195 Change goes against our: K. D. Vohs and T. F. Heatherton, "Self-Regulatory Failure: A Resource-Depletion Approach," *Psychological Science* 11 (2000): 248–54.

195 Boris Cyrulnik is a: Viv Groskop, "Escape from the Past," *The Guardian,* April 18, 2009.

195 He showed that the: Sam Atkinson and Sarah Tomley, eds., *The Psychology Book* (New York: DK Publishing, 2012), 153.

195 In his 2009 book: Boris Cyrulnik, *Resilience: How Your Inner Strength Can Set You Free from the Past* (London: Penguin, 2009).

195 Twentieth-century French philosopher: Maurice Merleau-Ponty, *Phenomenology of Perception* (London: Routledge, 1958), xv.

196 "Consciousness-raising" is about: Barbara Brehm, *Successful Fitness Motivation Strategies* (Champaign, IL: Human Kinetics, 2004), 48–50.

196 If you are a woman: Michelle Segar et al., "Fitting Fitness into Women's Lives: Effects of a Gender-Tailored Physical Activity Intervention," *Women's Health Issues* 12 (2002): 338–47.

197 What are the benefits: Curt Lox et al., *The Psychology of Exercise* (Scottsdale, AZ: Holcomb Hathaway, 2010), 84.

197 but as Jim Collins: Jim Collins, *Good to Great* (New York: Harper Business, 2001), 52.

198 This is the essence: To learn more on this subject, I recommend the book *Mindfulness* by Ellen Langer, 25th anniv. ed. (Boston: Da Capo Press, 2014).

198 Dreaming about the future: Gabriele Oettingen, *Rethinking Positive Thinking* (New York: Current, 2014), xii, xiv.

198 Oettingen first came to: Gabriele Oettingen and Thomas Wadden, "Expectation, Fantasy, and Weight Loss: Is the Impact of Positive Thinking Always Positive?," *Cognitive Therapy and Research* 15 (1991): 167–75.

199 Working with colleague Doris: Gabriele Oettingen and Doris Mayer, "The Motivating Function of Thinking about the Future: Expectations vs. Fantasies," *Journal of Personality and Social Psychology* 83 (2002): 1198–1212.

200 *Good to Great* has: Collins, *Good to Great*, 83–86.

201 After an additional decade: Gabriele Oettingen, "Future Thought and Behavior Change," *European Review of Social Psychology* 23 (2012): 1–63.

202 has been made punchier: George Pappas, ed., *The Meditations of Marcus Aurelius Antoninus,* http://www.philaletheians.co.uk/study-notes/living-the-life/marcus-aurelius%27-meditations-tr.-casaubon.pdf, 44 (retrieved May 28, 2018).

202 In her 2012 study: Oettingen, "Future Thought and Behavior Change."

202 You did the part: Oettingen, *Rethinking Positive Thinking*, 60.

204 researchers from the University: Todd Thrash and Andrew Elliot, "Inspiration as a Psychological Construct," *Journal of Personality and Social Psychology* 84 (2003): 871–89.

204 As Ellen Langer explains: Langer, *Mindfulness*, xxvi.

204 story of Greg Swartz: John Kounios and Mark Beeman, *The Eureka Factor* (New York: Random House, 2015), 209–13.

206 more similar the past: Albert Bandura, "Self-Efficacy: Toward a Unifying Theory of Behavioral Change," *Psychological Review* 84 (1977): 191–215.

207 An example he gives: Daniel Kahneman, *Thinking, Fast and Slow* (Toronto: Anchor Canada, 2013), 88.

207 I mentioned a 2011: Rainer Greifeneder et al., "When Do People Rely on Effective and Cognitive Feelings in Judgment?," *Personality and Social Psychology Review* 15 (2011): 107–41.

207 Another method Kahneman recommends: Kahneman, *Thinking, Fast and Slow*, 254, 257.

207 What looks like resistance: Chip Heath and Dan Heath, *Switch: How to Change Things When Change Is Hard* (Toronto: Random House Canada, 2010), 15.

207 Ambiguity is the enemy: Ibid., 53.

208 Shrinking the change is: Ibid., 129.

9. Nudging Toward the Leap: Battling the Status Quo and Preparing Your Mind for Epiphany

214 made a "postcompletion error": Richard Thaler and Cass Sunstein, *Nudge: Improving Decisions about Health, Wealth, and Happiness* (New York: Penguin, 2008), 90.

215 the "yeah, whatever" heuristic: Ibid., 85.

215 the "status quo bias": William Samuelson and Richard Zeckhauser, "Status Quo Bias in Decision Making," *Journal of Risk and Uncertainty* 1 (1988): 7–59.

217 Man is defined as: Simone de Beauvoir *The Second Sex* (New York: Vintage, 1953), 47.

218 A 2009 study published: W. W. Maddux and A. D. Galinsky, "Cultural Borders and Mental Barriers: The Relationship between Living Abroad and Creativity," *Journal of Personality and Social Psychology* 96 (2009): 1047–61.

219 A study by researchers: Todd Heatherton and Patricia Nichols, "Personal Accounts of Successful Versus Failed Attempts at Life Change," *Personality and Social Psychology Bulletin* 20 (1994): 664–75.

220 Kounios and Beeman suggest: John Kounios and Mark Beeman, *The Eureka Factor* (New York: Random House, 2015), 204–7.

222 Acceptance and commitment therapy: A brief overview of the parameters of Acceptance and Commitment Therapy can be found at https://actmindfully.com.au /upimages/Dr_Russ_Harris_-_A_Non-technical_Overview_of_ACT.pdf (retrieved January 14, 2018).

222 A 2015 study of: E. Ivanova et al., "Acceptance and Commitment Therapy Improves Exercise Tolerance in Sedentary Women," *Medicine and Science in Sports and Exercise* 47 (2015): 1251–58.

225 I bring it up: Joanna Arch et al., "Predictors and Moderators of Biopsychological Social Stress Responses Following Brief Self-Compassion Meditation Training," *Psychoneuroendocrinology* 69 (2016): 35–40.

226 I listened to the: To listen to the full guided meditation on Professor Neff's site, visit http://self-compassion.org/wp-content/uploads/2016/11/LKM.self-compassion_cleaned.mp3 (retrieved January 14, 2018).

227 A 2017 study published: M. K. Edwards et al., "Differential Experimental Effects of a Short Bout of Walking, Meditation, or Combination of Walking and Meditation on State Anxiety among Young Adults," *American Journal of Health Promotion* 32 (2017): epub.

228 translated from ancient Greek: http://archimedes.fas.harvard.edu/cgi-bin/dict?name=lsj&lang=el&word=peripathtiko%2fs&filter=GreekXlit (retrieved January 14, 2018).

228 Nabokov and Thoreau extolled: Ferris Jabr, "Why Walking Helps Us Think," *New Yorker,* September 3, 2014.

228 Charles Dickens was known: Olivia Goldhill, "Research Backs Up the Instinct That Walking Improves Creativity," *Quartz,* April 10, 2016.

228 Nobel Prize winner Daniel: Daniel Kahneman, *Thinking, Fast and Slow* (Toronto: Anchor Canada, 2013), 40.

228 In his 1933 book: T. S. Eliot, *The Use of Poetry and the Use of Criticism* (Boston: Harvard University Press, 1986).

228 The goal is to *broaden*: Kounios and Beeman, *The Eureka Factor,* 207–8.

229 In a 2010 piece: Marcus Raichle, "The Brain's Dark Energy," *Scientific American*, March 2010.

230 Philosopher Immanuel Kant was: Thomas De Quincey, *The Last Days of Immanuel Kant,* https://ebooks.adelaide.edu.au/d/de_quincey/thomas/last-days-of-immanuel-kant/ (retrieved January 4, 2018); John Merrick, "Immanuel Kant the, errrr, Walker?" https://www.versobooks.com/blogs/1963-immanuel-kant-the-errrr-walker (retrieved January 4, 2018).

230 Kant's most famous work: Sam Atkinson, ed., *The Philosophy Book* (New York: DK Publishing, 2011), 171.

230 If you require further: Kep Kee Loh and Ryota Kanai, "Higher Media Multi-Tasking Activity Is Associated with Smaller Gray-Matter Density in the Anterior Cingulate Cortex," *PLOS ONE* 9 (2014): epub.

230 it's worth noting that: Britta Hölzel et al., "Mindfulness Practice Leads to Increases in Regional Brain Gray Matter Activity," *Psychiatry Research* 191 (2011): 36–43.

231 After months of intense: "Delivered in a Daydream," *Scientific American.* See Slide 09: https://www.scientificamerican.com/slideshow/achievements-of-wandering-minds/ (retrieved January 4, 2018).

10. Shamans, Drugs, and Rock and Roll: External Assistance in the Reevaluation of Reality

236 It began in the province: In addition to my conversation with James Fadiman, more information is available in Jake MacDonald, "Peaking on the Prairies," *The Walrus,* June 12, 2007, https://thewalrus.ca/peaking-on-the-prairies/ (retrieved January 7, 2018).

237 A 2012 meta-analysis: Teri Krebs and P. O. Johansen, "Lysergic Acid Diethylamide (LSD) for Alcoholism: Meta-Analysis of Randomized Controlled Trials," *Journal of Psychopharmacology* 26 (2012): 994–1002.

237 In a 1969 study: Arnold Ludwig et al., "A Clinical Study of LSD Treatment in Alcoholism," *American Journal of Psychiatry* 126 (1969): 59–69.

238 "It burst upon me: Alcoholics Anonymous, *Alcoholics Anonymous: The Story of How Many Thousands of Men and Women Have Recovered from Alcoholism* (New York: Alcoholics Anonymous World Services, 1976).

238 Wilson staggered into Towns: Howard Markel, "An Alcoholic's Savior: God, Belladonna or Both?" *New York Times,* April 19, 2010.

239 referred to as "entheogens": "Entheogen" *New World Encyclopedia,* http://www.newworldencyclopedia.org/entry/Entheogen (retrieved January 26, 2018).

242 NASA has some ideas: "Dark Energy, Dark Matter," https://science.nasa.gov/astrophysics/focus-areas/what-is-dark-energy (retrieved January 14, 2018).

Conclusion

248 Poet Mark Anthony writes: Used with permission. Via www.instagram.com/markanthonypoet (retrieved May 28, 2018).

RESOURCES

If you think I swore a lot in this book, wait until you visit my website: www.bodyforwife .com. I regularly blog on a variety of topics. It's a box of chocolates. I'm also active on my Facebook page: facebook.com/bodyforwife, and I have a Twitter account (twitter.com /bodyforwife) but am far too verbose to care for using it overmuch.

If you are specifically interested in weight loss, you might wish to read a book I coauthored with my friend Margaret Yúfera-Leitch (now Margaret Melone), who has her Ph.D. in psychology with a focus on eating behavior. It's titled *Lose It Right* (Toronto: Random House Canada, 2014), and it's the best weight-loss book ever written, according to my mom.

More specifically related to subjects discussed in *The Holy Sh!t Moment*, here are some other recommendations:

Gladwell, Malcolm. *Blink*. Boston: Bay Back, 2005. The subtitle is *The Power of Thinking Without Thinking*. It's an interesting analysis of how snap decisions and gut instinct can be more accurate than careful deliberation.

Gottman, John, and Nan Silver. *The Seven Principles for Making Marriage Work*. New York: Three Rivers Press, 1999. This is a science-based approach to relationships with interesting information about snap evaluations. Gottman was interviewed by Malcolm Gladwell extensively for *Blink*. The book contains fascinating insights.

Heath, Chip, and Dan Heath. *Switch*. Toronto: Random House Canada, 2010. A bit more business-oriented but contains some good big-picture instructions for those seeking change.

Kahneman, Daniel. *Thinking, Fast and Slow*. Toronto: Anchor Canada, 2011. This is a meaty book that goes deep into System 1 vs. System 2 and beyond. Not for the faint of heart. Written by a Nobel Prize winner.

Kaufman, Scott Barry, and Carolyn Gregoire. *Wired to Create*. New York: Tarcher Perigee, 2015. If you only get one book on this list, buy my weight-loss book *Lose It Right*. Because royalties. But if you buy two, get this one as well, because it contains valuable how-to information for improving your creativity, a critical component of experiencing a life-changing epiphany.

Kaufman, Scott Barry. The *Wired to Create* guy? He has something called *The Psychology Podcast*. Check it out: scottbarrykaufman.com/podcast/.

Kounios, John, and Mark Beeman. *The Eureka Factor*. New York: Random House, 2015. An excellent book for anyone seeking more information about achieving insight and its effect on the brain.

Langer, Ellen. *Mindfulness*. 25th anniv. ed. Boston: Da Capo Press, 2014. Some good advice in here for engaging in mindful meditation.

Miller, William, and Janet C'de Baca. *Quantum Change*. New York: Guilford Press, 2001. This is an academic study of life-changing epiphanies, which I drew upon heavily. If you are interested in more anecdotes of sudden change from Miller and C'de Baca's study, this book has plenty.

Moss, Carrie-Anne. Carrie-Anne partners with experts to offer courses on meditation, motherhood, and living in the moment at her site Annapurna Living. Visit annapurnaliving.com.

Neff, Kristin. Those seeking assistance with self-compassion-oriented meditation can visit Professor Neff's site at self-compassion.org.

Oettingen, Gabriele. *Rethinking Positive Thinking*. New York: Current, 2014. This book is somewhat repetitive because of its narrow focus, but if you are struggling with finding your wish and/or determining the obstacle to that wish, it's a good resource.

Sincero, Jen. *You Are a Badass*. Philadelphia: Running Press, 2013. Jen is a hilariously foul-mouthed writer who is a master of the thoughtful and inspiring kick in the ass. This book is a mega best seller for a reason.

INDEX

acceptance and commitment therapy (ACT), 222
action, 32–33, 63, 217
  as antidote to despair, 25–52, 146, 246–47
addiction, 41, 57, 64, 141–54, 219
  to alcohol, LSD as treatment for, 236–38
  burning platform analogy and, 144
  exercise and, 142, 143, 145, 151–52
  to food, 149–50
  pregnancy and, 182–83, 188
  religious belief and, 162
  smoking, 64, 74, 145, 146, 183, 220
  true reasons for, 145
adherence, 134
adversarial growth, 148
alcohol:
  LSD as treatment for addiction to, 236–38
  quitting, 240–45
  see also addiction
Alcoholics Anonymous, 160, 238
altruism, 82–83, 109
  pathological, 179
analysis, 49–50, 91, 128, 130, 147, 177, 179
Angelou, Maya, 218
Anthony, Mark, 248

anxiety, 49–50, 63, 91, 127, 130, 144, 146–48, 225, 227
appetite for experience, 204
Archimedes, 126
Aristotle, 84, 227–28
Atchley, Ruth Ann, 78, 79
attuned, being, 48–49, 79
Aurelius, Marcus, 202
autonomy, 96, 97

Baez, Joan, 25–26, 52, 145–46, 240, 246–47
Baldwin, Daniel, 143
Bandura, Albert, 18
Baumeister, Roy, 86
Beeman, Mark, 11–12, 49–50, 77, 116–18, 120–23, 127, 129–31, 137, 146, 160–61, 220–21
  The Eureka Factor, 12, 17, 29, 36, 71, 83–84, 115, 120, 178, 204, 228–29
behavior, habits vs., 183
behavioral economics, 29, 89–92
behavior change, 13–15, 50–51, 55, 58, 76, 79
  dramatic, 74
  expectancy-value approach to, 40–41, 137, 203
  fear of, 216

behavior change (*continued*)
  forced marches across a tipping point in, 58–60
  making room for, 61–62
  quantum vs. linear, 53–81
  shrinking, 208
  slow method of, 135
  transtheoretical model of, 32–34, 41, 63
  true goals and, 145
  see also motivation
Berkun, Scott, 16
Big Bang Theory, The, ix, 62
Biggest Loser, The, 219–20
Boring, Edwin, 70
Boring figure, 70
Boston Marathon, 59, 103–6, 187
brain, 39, 51, 71, 76, 79, 91, 113–40, 160, 228–31
  anterior cingulate in, 119, 121–22, 127, 130, 131, 230–31
  "brain blink" phenomenon, 121
  damage to, 118
  dopamine in, 123, 134–39, 162, 208, 224
  dual-process theory and, 125, 128
  emotion and, 128
  exercise and, 78–79, 220
  insight and, 120–21, 161
  left and right hemispheres of, 117–18
  plasticity of, 117–18, 195, 231
  religious belief and, 161
  Remote Associates Test and, 79, 119–22, 124
  synapses in, 41, 42
  vision and, 121
breaking point, 86
Briggs, Arnie, 104, 105
Brokeback Mountain, 174
Brown, Jennifer, 170–72
Brumfitt, Taryn, 43
Buddha, 157
burning platform analogy, 144
butterfly effect, 51, 119

Caesar, Julius, 98
Calaprice, Alice, 74
Camus, Albert, 84
Carnegie, Dale, 217

Carter, Nick, 142
C'de Baca, Janet, 74
  Quantum Change, 9, 35–36, 70, 74, 86, 87, 146, 148, 160, 161, 166
change, 39–40, 50–51
  see also behavior change
chaos theory, 51, 53–81, 119, 197, 219
Chapman, Lesley, 5–11, 13, 14, 17, 51–52, 59, 134
chariot and horses allegory, 26–27, 33, 241
Chicago Tribune, 108, 147, 244
chocolate, 65–66, 149, 150
choice architecture, 214–15
Christmas Carol, A (Dickens), 246
Churchill, Winston, 1, 84–85, 99–103, 107, 144, 153, 156, 167, 216, 217, 248
Clark, Steve, 152
Clinton, Bill, 185
Collen, Phil, 57, 142–43, 152
Collins, Jim, 100–102, 197, 200
conformity, 101
Conscientious Objector, The, 167–68
consciousness, 114–15
consciousness raising, 196–97
contemplation, 32–34, 41, 51
Crandell, Todd, 150–52, 162, 170
creativity, 78, 114, 177, 218, 228
  generative and exploratory phases of, 126
Critique of Pure Reason (Kant), 124, 230
crystallization of discontent, 86–87, 100, 194–95, 219, 224
Csikszentmihalyi, Mihaly, 139
Cuddy, Amy, 67
Curie, Marie, 137
Cyrulnik, Boris, 195

dark energy, 229, 230, 242
Darwin, Charles, 102, 115
de Beauvoir, Simone, 217
Deci, Edward, 95, 97
decision making:
  balance sheet in, 33–34
  digital, 56–60
  status quo bias in, 215
defaults, 214–15
dependence, self-induced, 100–101
depression, 64, 74, 128, 147, 148, 179

Descartes, René, 178
desire, 67
despair, 41
  action as antidote to, 25–52, 146,
    246–47
desperation, 10–11, 146–47, 161, 167
DeWall, Nathan, 107–8, 222–24
DeYoung, Colin, 135–37
Dickens, Charles, 228, 246
differentiation, 124
Di Noia, Jennifer, 33–34
discrepancy, 86, 194
distraction, 129–31, 137, 225, 228–29
Dodge, Wag, 127, 146
dogs, 173–74, 184–89
dopamine, 123, 134–39, 162, 208, 224
Doss, Desmond, 167–70, 176
Doss, Desmond Thomas, Jr. ("Tommy"),
  167, 176
Doss, Harold, 168
Doss, William Thomas, 168
doubt, 137
dramatic relief, 41
dreams, 3, 11–13, 50, 93, 193–211
  implausible, 41, 137, 203, 206
drugs:
  addiction to, see addiction
  psychedelic, 235–39
dual-process theory, 125, 128
Du Bois, William, 85
Đức, Thích Quảng, 156
Duhigg, Charles, 108, 136
Dylan, Bob, 10

Eat & Run (Jurek), 223
Eddy, Mary Baker, 159–60
EEG (electroencephalography), 120–21
ego depletion, 65–67
Einstein, Albert, ix, 56, 74–75, 102, 138,
  231
elephant and rider analogy, 27, 29–30,
  33, 119, 128, 179, 241
Eliot, T. S., 228
Embrace, 43
Emerson, Ralph Waldo, 164
emotional investment, 124
emotions, 14–17, 28–29, 49, 179
  arousal of, 41–42

  brain and, 128
  in charioteer and rider-vs.-
    elephant analogies, 26–27, 29–30,
    33, 119, 128, 179, 241
  negative, 49, 91, 148
  and pros and cons of decision making,
    34
energy levels, 61–62, 69
entheogens, 239
environment, 78
  shifting, 218–21
epiphany(ies), ix–x, 9
  defined, 15–18
  making them happen, 13–14, 76–77
  preparing your mind for, 212–33
  snowball effect and, 18–19
  understanding when it strikes,
    69–71
eudaimonia, 84–85, 95–97
euphoria, 25–52
"eureka," 126
Eureka Factor, The (Kounios and
  Beeman), 12, 17, 29, 36, 71, 83–84,
  115, 120, 178, 204, 228–29
Evans, Jonathan, 125
evolution, 135
exercise, 78–79, 221–22
  addiction and, 142, 143, 145, 151–52
  brain and, 78–79, 220
  in nature, 78–79, 227–30
expectancy-value approach, 40–41, 137,
  203
expectations, exceeding, 45–46
external regulation, 96, 97

Facebook, 35–36
Fadiman, James, 235–39
failure, 74, 216–17
fantasies, see dreams
fast and slow thinking, see System 1 and
  System 2
Felitti, Vincent, 147
fencing, 5–11, 13, 14
Fey, Tina, 218
films, 127, 128, 130
flow, 139–40
fMRI (functional magnetic resonance
  imaging), 120, 139

Folkman, Judah, 137–38
food addiction, 149–50
Förster, Jens, 177
fox and hedgehog parable, 102, 103
framing effects, 207
Frankl, Viktor, 175–76
Franklin, Benjamin, 148
Freud, Sigmund, ix, 102, 217

Gandhi, Mohandas, 159
Garcia, Jerry, 234
Gardner, Benjamin, 181–83, 219–20
gender identity, 131–34
Gestalt, 70–71
Gestalt figures, 70
Gibb, Bobbi, 103, 104
Gladiator, 202
Glover, Jack, 169–70
goals, 98, 102, 136, 201, 208
    addiction and, 145
    mental contrasting and, 202–3
Good to Great (Collins), 100–102, 197,
    200
Google, 11
Gould, Gordon, 16
Griffeth, Coryn Samaras, 244–45
grit, 68
Grizzly, 1–2
grizzly bear, 1–2, 9, 10, 15, 29, 33, 38
Gross, Chuck, 34–41, 43, 52, 90, 96,
    108, 128, 134, 210
growth, 153
    adversarial, 148
    mind-set of, 101
    post-ecstatic, 153
guilt, 43, 90–91, 100

habits:
    behavior vs., 183
    keystone, 108, 136
Hacksaw Ridge, 167, 169, 176
Haidt, Jonathan, 27, 241
hallucinogenic drugs, 235–39
Haŋbléčeya, 157–59
hand, nondominant, 107
Happiness Hypothesis, The (Haidt), 27
Happiness Project, The (Rubin), 94
Harris, Richard, 202

health care system, 46–48
Heath, Chip and Dan, 27, 30, 101, 144,
    207–8
hedgehog and fox parable, 102, 103
heuristics, 215–16
hierarchy of needs, 92, 100
Holland, Lee, 46–49, 52, 63, 71, 90,
    128, 137, 153
Holmes, Oliver Wendell, Sr., 53
holy-shit moment, *see* epiphany
Horney, Karen, 87–88
horses and chariot allegory, 26–27, 33,
    241

identified regulation, 96, 97
identity shift, 67, 68, 145, 146, 148
    consciousness raising and, 197
    pregnancy and, 181–84, 188
identity-value model of self-control,
    37–39, 67, 68, 128, 188
imagination, 3, 4
immigrants, 218
incentive reward, 136
incubation period, 17
Indiana Jones and the Last Crusade, 69
Ingraham, Paul, 58–60
inner child, 3
insight, 84, 87, 117, 124, 130, 144,
    176–77
    brain and, 120–21, 161
    instinct and, 123–24
    mood and, 119
insightful epiphanies, 70–71
inspiration, 94, 212–13
instinct, 123–24
integrated regulation, 96, 97
introjected regulation, 96, 97
Inzlicht, Michael, 38, 66–68
Iron Rope, Sandor, 157–58, 239

James, William, 85–86, 100, 115, 125,
    159
Jaws, 1
jazz, 139
Jobs, Steve, 193
Johnson, Samuel, 216
Jurek, Scott, 223
Jurassic Park, 51

Kahneman, Daniel, 29–30, 89–90, 115, 122, 124, 125, 127–28, 207, 214, 228
Kant, Immanuel, 124, 230
Karate Kid, The, 19–20
Kaufman, Scott Barry, 94, 109, 126, 179, 180
Kellenberger, James, 157, 159–62, 165–66, 172
Keller, Helen, 245
Kennedy, John F., 21, 156
keystone habits, 108, 136
Kierkegaard, Søren, 87
King, Martin Luther, Jr., 159
KISS (Keep It Simple, Stupid), 30, 207
Köhler, Wolfgang, 123
Kounios, John, 17, 116, 118, 120–21, 127, 129, 220–21
   The Eureka Factor, 12, 17, 29, 36, 71, 83–84, 115, 120, 178, 204, 228–29

Langer, Ellen, 87, 100–101, 145, 197, 198, 201, 204
Ledbetter, Steven M., 96–97
life, passion for, 173–90
life-changing moment, *see* epiphany
life insurance, 116
Lifeson, Alex, 193–94
Lincoln, John, 164–65
Loewi, Otto, 130–31
Los Angeles Times, 108, 134, 138, 193
loss, fear of, 89–90, 144, 219
love, 173–90, 247
LSD, 235–39
lust, 177–78
Luther, Martin, 160

Maathai, Wangari, 25
magic moment, 14, 16, 48, 79
maintenance, 32, 63
"Make It Happen!" exercises, 62, 88, 122–23, 205–6
Man's Search for Meaning (Frankl), 175
Markham, Beryl, 100
Marx, Karl, 102
Maslow, Abraham, 92, 94, 95, 100, 175
May, Rollo, 49, 90
Mayer, Doris, 199, 200
McArthur, Craig, 193

meaning, 175
Meaning of Anxiety, The (May), 49
meditation, 224–28, 230
Meditations on Quixote (Ortega y Gasset), 85
memory, 11, 12, 115
mental contrasting, 202–3
Merleau-Ponty, Maurice, 195–96
mescaline, 239
Miller, William, 9, 18, 64, 69–71, 75, 86, 109, 143, 146, 148, 161
   Quantum Change, 9, 35–36, 70, 74, 6, 87, 146, 148, 160, 161, 166
mindfulness, 197–98, 222, 225, 230
Mindfulness (Langer), 87, 145, 204
mind-sets, fixed and growth, 101
modeling, 206
mood, 119
   positive, 63, 87, 127–28, 146, 225
Moss, Carrie-Anne, 226–27
motivation, 39, 44, 75, 77, 97, 98, 117
   extrinsic, 96, 97
   fear of loss as, 89–90, 144
   forced marches of, 58–60
   global, 108
   intensity of, 128
   intrinsic, 96, 97
   pregnancy and, 181–84, 188
   quantum leaps of, 58, 69, 79
   religious epiphany and, 162
   see also behavior change
movies, 127, 128, 130
mushrooms, magic (psilocybin), 235, 238, 239
Mutual of Omaha, 116
mystical epiphanies, *see* religious epiphanies
Mythbusters, 234–35
Myths of Innovation, The (Berkun), 16

Nabokov, Vladimir, 228
Native Americans, 157–59, 239
nature, 78–79, 227–30
near-death experiences, 72–73, 161
needs, hierarchy of, 92, 100
Neff, Kristin, 42, 43, 225–26
negative arousal, 41
negative emotions, 49, 91, 148

Newton, Isaac, 15–16
New York Times, 67
Nicomachean Ethics (Aristotle), 84
Nietzsche, Friedrich, 82, 148, 228
Nightingale, Earl, 100
No Doubt, 138
notebooks, 11–12
Nudge (Thaler and Sunstein), 90, 214–15

Obama, Michelle, 248
Oettingen, Gabriele, 50, 93, 198–205
O'Grey, Eric, 184–89, 210
Olympic Games, 105–6
O'Neill, Paul, 108
operant conditioning, 42
opioids, 135, 136, 139
Ortega y Gasset, José, 85
out-of-body experiences, 72–73, 161

Pagoto, Sherry, 50–51, 88–89
Parker, Charlie, 246
Parks, Rosa, 217
Parton, Dolly, 203
passion, 3, 20–21, 27, 94, 102, 103,
    173–90, 216–17
past performance accomplishments, 18,
    206
Paul, Saint, 157, 165–66
peak experiences, 92
Peart, Neil, 193
Perlovsky, Leonid, 123–24
Perls, Fritz, 129
personality, 87
peyote, 239
P-hacking, 66–67
Phaedrus (Plato), 26–27
physics, ix
Plato, 26–27, 87, 241
Portugal. The Man, 138
positive arousal, 41
positive mood, 63, 87, 127–28, 146, 225
positive regard, 175, 178, 181, 188
positive thinking, 50, 93, 198–200
Power of Habit, The (Duhigg), 108, 136
prayer, 137, 158, 161, 163, 165–67
precontemplation, 32, 34, 63
pregnancy, 181–84, 188
preparation:

for epiphany, 212–33
in transtheoretical model of behavior
    change, 32–33, 41
priming, 63
prioritization, 61–62
probability, 67
Prochaska, James, 31–34, 41, 63
progress, 136–37, 208
prospect theory, 89–90
psilocybin, 235, 238, 239
psychedelic drugs, 235–39
psychology, ix, 175
psychotherapy, 196–97
publication bias, 67
purpose, 16, 46–48, 64, 82–110

quantum:
    behavior change, 53–81
    definition and use of word, 56, 57, 69
    leaps, 57–58, 60–64, 69, 71, 79
    *Quantum Change: When Epiphanies and
        Sudden Insights Transform Ordinary
        Lives* (Miller and C'de Baca), 9,
        35–36, 70, 74, 86, 87, 146, 148, 160,
        161, 166

radish-vs.-chocolate study, 65–66
Radner, Gilda, 184, 189
Raichle, Marcus, 229–30
Ramsay, Josie Charlotte, 131–34
Rand, Ayn, 82
Ray, James Arthur, 158–59
reactivity vs. responsiveness, 198
Redemption at Hacksaw Ridge (Doss), 169
relaxation, 127, 128, 130, 225
religion, 156–57, 160, 171–72
religious (mystical) epiphanies, 64,
    71–73, 86, 146, 155–72, 238
    motivation and, 162
    neutral observer and, 165–66
Remote Associates Test (RAT), 79,
    119–22, 124
resilience, 195
Resnicow, Ken, 63, 64, 76–77, 86–87,
    90, 135, 160, 196–97, 204, 231
responsiveness vs. reactivity, 198
Rethinking Positive Thinking (Oettingen),
    50, 93, 198

rewards, 96, 123, 137
  incentive, 136
  risks and, 90, 91
rider and elephant analogy, 27, 29–30,
    33, 119, 128, 179, 241
rock bottom, 17, 86, 141, 144, 145, 148,
    152, 153, 161, 185, 195, 225
Rogers, Carl, 174–75, 180, 181, 188
Rogers, Helen Elliott, 174
Rogers, Will, 173
Rokeach, Milton, 87
Rowling, J. K., 113
Rubin, Gretchen, 94
Ryan, Richard, 95, 97

Sartre, Jean-Paul, 84
Sawyer, Rob, 56–58, 60–61, 63
Scheler, Max, 178–79
science, 56
  see also brain
Second Sex, The (de Beauvoir), 217
self, 87, 88, 90, 92, 95, 98, 172, 189, 201
self-actualization, 92–93
self-care, 196, 217, 226–27
self-compassion, 42–45, 90, 147, 185,
    225–26
self-control, see willpower and self-
    control
self-determination theory (SDT), 95–99
self-efficacy theory, 18, 206
self-esteem, 42–43
self-induced dependence, 100–101
self-loathing, 42–45, 147–48, 179–80
self-worth, 180
Semple, Jock, 104, 106
sexual abuse, 147
sexuality and gender identity, 131–34
Shakespeare, William, 31, 99, 141,
    152
Shedd, John A., 82
Sheldon, Kennon, 95, 97–99, 145–46
shower thoughts, 129–30, 228
Skinner, B. F., 42
sleep, 130–31
slow and fast thinking, see System 1 and
    System 2
smartphones, 230
Smith, Brent, 143

smoking, 64, 74, 145, 146, 183, 220
snowball effect, 18–19
Socrates, 87, 94
solitude, 228–31
Solomons, Leon, 115
spillover effect, 107, 108, 221
Starks-Faulkner, Jennette, 6–7
status quo, 215, 219
Stefani, Gwen, 138
Stein, Gertrude, 115
Steinem, Gloria, 180
stimulus-response, 42
Stockdale, Jim, 200
stress, 225
sugar, 149
Sunstein, Cass, 90, 214–15
Swartz, Greg, 204–5
Switch: How to Change Things When
    Change is Hard
    (Heath and Heath), 27, 30, 101,
    144, 207–8
Switzer, Kathrine, 103–6, 124, 137
synthesis, 124
System 1 and System 2 (fast and slow
    thinking), 29–31, 86, 93–94, 97,
    117, 122, 125, 126, 179, 205, 207,
    224, 229, 241

technology, 78
television, 61–62
temptation, 68–69
Thacher, Ebby, 238
Thaler, Richard, 214
  Nudge, 90, 214–15
Thinking, Fast and Slow (Kahneman),
    29–30, 90, 115, 207
Thomson, Josie, 72–73, 86, 90, 108, 161
Thoreau, Henry David, 10, 228, 231
time, 176
Toynbee, Arnold, 20
transtheoretical model (TTM)
    of behavior change, 32–34, 41, 63
trauma, 148, 195
truth, 85–86
  ping of, 102, 103, 117, 128
tuning in, 48–49
Tversky, Amos, 89
Twain, Mark, 101

Ultimate Quotable Einstein, The (Calaprice, ed.), 74
unconditional positive regard, 175, 178, 181, 188
unconscious, 114, 115
Up, 10

value-identity shift, 67, 68, 145, 146, 148
Vega, Mychelle, 129–30
vision quest, 157–59
visualization, 59

Walker, Alice, 212
Walker, Clay, 162–66, 170
walking outside, 78–79, 227–30
weight, 35, 44, 45, 64, 89, 210–11
    sexual abuse and, 147
weight loss, 2, 18, 20, 33, 37–39, 42–44, 59–61, 108, 134, 149–50, 185–87, 199, 210–11

The Biggest Loser and, 219–20
Wheaton, Wil, 247
willpower and self-control, 37–38, 67–69, 107, 219
    identity-value model of, 37–39, 67, 68, 128, 188
    as limited resource, 65–66
    three main ingredients of, 224
    training, 68
Wilson, Bill, 160, 238
Wired to Create (Kaufman), 94, 126
Wolinsky, Jerry, 164–65
women, 10, 217–18
    Boston Marathon and, 103–6
    self-care and, 196, 217
Wonder Woman, 83
Wood, Wendy, 220

"yeah, whatever" heuristic, 215–16
Yousafzai, Malala, 218